MIND THE GAP

Dr Karen Gurney is a highly specialized clinical psychologist and certified psychosexologist, and a recognized national expert in the theory and practice of therapy around all aspects of sexual well-being and function. She is currently Lead Psychosexual Therapist at 56 Dean Street (Chelsea and Westminster Hospital NHS Foundation Trust), as well as Director of the Havelock Clinic, an independent sexual problems service based in Harley Street and in the City of London. Dr Gurney has written for and been featured in publications such as *Marie Claire, Cosmopolitan* and *Refinery29*. She has appeared on BBC2's *Victoria Derbyshire* show and is the expert attached to Cherry Healey, Lisa Williams and Anniki Sommerville's podcast, The Hotbed Collective (@thehotbedcollective), regularly appearing in their live shows and podcasts. She is also an ambassador for www.thepornconversation.org – a not-for-profit initiative set up by Erika Lust designed to help parents and carers talk to young people about porn use. Dr Gurney is on Instagram as @thesexdoctor. *Mind The Gap* is her first book.

MIND THE GAP

The truth about desire, and how to futureproof your sex life

Dr Karen Gurney

First published in 2020 by HEADLINE HOME
An imprint of HEADLINE PUBLISHING GROUP

15

Cataloguing in Publication Data is available from the British Library

ISBN 978 1 4722 6713 9

Diagrams by Louise Turpin

Typeset in Dante MT and Futura by Avon DataSet Ltd,
Bidford-on-Avon, Warwickshire

Printed and bound in Great Britain by Clays Ltd, Elcograf S.p.A.

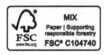

Headline's policy is to use papers that are natural, renewable and
recyclable products and made from wood grown in sustainable forests.
The logging and manufacturing processes are expected to conform
to the environmental regulations of the country of origin.

HEADLINE PUBLISHING GROUP
An Hachette UK Company
Carmelite House
50 Victoria Embankment
London EC4Y 0DZ

The authorised representative in the EEA is Hachette Ireland, 8 Castlecourt
Centre, Dublin 15, D15 XTP3, Ireland (email: info@hbgi.ie)

www.headline.co.uk
www.hachette.co.uk

Contents

Two
The Truth About Sex and Desire

Three
How to Futureproof Your Sex Life, for Life

Introduction

What if I told you that everything you've been led to believe about your own sexuality wasn't true? That the standards you've been judging yourself and your sex life by, and often feeling you're failing at, are unrealistic for most of us and cannot be realized? That it's possible to simultaneously feel little or no spontaneous desire in your sexual relationship, but also have a happy and mutually satisfying sex life long term?

It might well be hard to believe.

There aren't many areas of science where we have got it so wrong for so long that gross inaccuracy has seeped into our collective psyche, but sex is one of them. Sex is an area where so much of our understanding comes from culture, folklore, religion, hearsay and magazines that we have lost track of the facts. We are too blinded by the pervasive and all-encompassing impact of this cultural and social story to see clearly.

My professional life as a clinical psychologist and psychosexologist in this field has been spent unlearning everything I thought I knew about people and sex in order to be able to help the people who come to see me in therapy. I spend a great deal of time working with women and their partners in therapy sessions around the issue of dissatisfaction with a sex life that, to them (or their partners), isn't quite hitting the mark. A sex life where the desire they feel for one another is not as present as they feel it should be, and this seems like a looming, impending disaster in their lives.

The reality is that they – us, we – have been sold a lie. Sex science has made some surprising discoveries in the last few decades, since it first brought forward ideas about how human desire worked, ideas that came to dominate popular opinion and society and shape how we understand our own sex lives. What came later were new understandings and ideas that have revolutionized the field of sex therapy even further, but this knowledge has not yet trickled its way down from academia or therapists to the mainstream, so the old ideas remain and hang over our sex lives like a sword of Damocles of impossible standards.

But why? Surely, if it's that important, people would be talking about it? Well, sadly, the evidence of history shows 'real' facts about sex and sexuality often struggle to cut through the thick fog of moral, social and cultural opinion. You only have to look at other areas of sex science to see it. Ideas about masturbation making you go blind, which were prevalent in the early nineteenth century, are still brought to the therapy room to this day. The belief that monogamy 'works', despite evidence that, for many humans, it can be challenging, is rooted in the institutions of culture and religion, rather than any scientific evidence demonstrating that humans were made to stick with one partner for life. And, lastly (and possibly, to you, most importantly), that you should feel sexual desire randomly and frequently for your long-term sexual partner, that good sex should 'just happen', and that this desire should prompt you to have sex whenever the whim takes you.

Take a second to reflect on this. At this current moment in time, do you believe these ideas? Ideas such as, in your sexual relationships, you should frequently and spontaneously desire sex with your partner? It would surprise me if you don't believe it strongly (even if it's not happening for you). Everything we have been led to believe speaks to this idea. Films, TV and music perpetuate it. Everyone is worried about how much sex they are having (and that it's not enough), and a relationship that can stand the test of time and *still* be passionate is the holy grail for most people. But, ironically, there's another discourse that sits alongside all this. A warning bound up with jokes and innuendo (especially related to marriage), that it's impossible to have a happy sex life in a long-term relationship. That couples who commit to each other basically throw away any hope of ever having good sex for the long term, but that, somehow, long-term companionship should make up for this.

So which is it? Should we be expecting passion that lasts a lifetime or sex only on birthdays after the honeymoon period?

There are problems inherent in both of these ideas. In the first, an impossible ideal of everlasting passion that can somehow endure all manner of relationship dissatisfaction, life events and changes to our bodies and our identities, without any conscious effort. In the second, a sense of hopeless inevitability that sex is doomed and that it can never be resolved, no matter how hard you try: a kind of passion black hole.

The truth is that great sex is cultivated, not ever present, but we need to understand how desire works and develop knowledge and skills regarding how to cultivate it. And those tropes we mentioned? Of everlasting unwavering passion with little effort? Or of long-term relationships inevitably moving forward to total sexlessness? Neither of them help us one bit.

The title of this book, *Mind The Gap*, makes reference to the differences between how we think our sex lives should be (often based on unhelpful comparisons) and how our sex lives *actually* are, as well as the difference between what we need to know about sex and desire to have great sex and what most of us *actually* know. There are also other gaps which influence our sex lives negatively and which will feature in this book. Some of which you will probably be familiar with already, such as gaps in gender equality (yes, inequality affects our sex lives too), and others which you may have heard of, such as the orgasm gap (where women, particularly straight women, have less pleasure during sexual encounters with men than the men they are having sex with). My hope is that reading this book will help you close these gaps in your own life and relationships.

Couples who come to see me for therapy in regards to desire often hint in the first session that they expect the work that we will need to do to be long and arduous. As I hope you will learn from this book, the reality is far from this, and the process can even be as quick as a realization that might happen in a single session (or on one page), or a few sessions (chapters). The harder work, in fact – if there is any – can sometimes be the unravelling of patterns that have formed, which then also need to be addressed, so as not to under-mine this new way of seeing things. In this book this aspect will be addressed with useful exercises I've set out at the end of each relevant chapter for you to try.

I'm hoping that you picked up this book because you can see the potential for a more satisfying sex life. The truth is, all of us can, and should, strive for our sex life to get better and better over time. If you find this hard to believe, you have fallen for the societal myth we talked about earlier – that sex declines in a relationship over time.

This book is for all women (or female identifying people) of any age. This doesn't mean that this information isn't also of use to those identifying as men or non-binary (in fact, much of the content will be equally relatable), but rather that we'll be focusing on the enormous influence of gender on sexuality, and so the content might speak more to those whose gender identity is female. When I refer to women throughout this book, I mean all women, no matter what sex they were assigned at birth. That said, there are key differences in the experience of sex for trans and non-binary people, related to society, culture, transitioning, being on gender-affirming hormones or having had lower surgery, which I will not be addressing here.

If you are in a sexual relationship with a woman, this book is for you too, as you will learn information about your partner's desire that will change the way you understand your sex life. This book is relevant for women of all sexualities, and you will find information related to the key differences in how the gender identity of your partner(s) might influence your current sex life as the book continues. There are many similarities between the sex lives of women who have sex with women and women who have sex with men, but also some key differences, which provide key insights for all of us about how we can better understand our sex lives.

When I refer to sex, what I have in mind is not a narrow definition of one sexual act, such as penetrative vaginal sex, as is often the meaning of 'sex' in our society. In fact, I'm not assuming what sex means to you at all. This is partly the journey, understanding what 'sex' is about for us, which is in constant flux, and then basing our current sexual lives on this understanding, not someone else's blueprint. I also do not see 'good sex' as just the absence of a sexual problem. Let's aspire to more than that, shall we?

My hope is that it will give you a new sense of what's 'normal'. It may lead you to the conclusion that you were expecting something impossible of yourself and your sex life in every long-term relationship that you've been in so far, but it will also give you a comprehensive understanding of how desire *really* works, so that you can be in the driving seat of how you'd like desire to feature in your sex life over the course of the rest of your life. No longer a passive recipient, but in control of the direction you want it to go and the destination you are aspiring to.

Part One will give you a brief overview of the social, cultural and political history to where we find ourselves right now. Chapter 1 will cover how institutions such as science, religion, psychology, psychiatry and the media have authored different bits of this story, each with their own objectives and biases. This is an important backdrop to many of the subsequent chapters. In Chapter 2 we'll learn the real facts about what's happening in the sex lives of the UK population and across the world – how much sex are people *really* having? What kind of sex? How many of those people are dissatisfied or worried about desire? Then, in Chapter 3, we'll talk anatomy, orgasms, sex education and understanding what your individual 'conditions for good sex' are. Part One is about understanding the forces that have led to the way you think and feel about your sex life right now.

In Part Two we'll be opening up and exploring some of the key aspects of how sex and desire work. This will include the impact of society on how we understand and act sexually, how the context of our relationships help or hinder our sex lives, and how our brains process and facilitate sex and desire. I'll also be introducing you to more recent understandings of how desire actually works. This new understanding will give you a clearer idea of the changes you can make in your own relationship to have better sex and nurture desire.

In the final section, Part Three, we'll take all of this forward and build on it. How can we put all we've learned into practice and make the changes we now realize we need to make with a partner? What other aspects of our relationships should we work on if we want to keep the sex hot? How do we keep a sex life on track despite the sudden onslaught of new life challenges, or over time? Put simply, how do we futureproof our sex life, for life?

I wrote this book for two reasons. One is to disseminate information about sex that I feel all women should know. The second reason is because I have seen first-hand the difference that this kind of perspective can make to people's sex lives and relationship satisfaction. I hope it's the change you're looking for right now.

Ready?

Let's start a revolution.

One

Common Misconceptions and How They are Holding Us Back

1
A brief history of sex, science and gender politics

How did we get here?

It would be impossible to write a book on women's sexuality and desire without outlining some of the key social, political and scientific influences that led us to where we are today. As you read through this book, you will discover that desire exists within a constraining framework of gender politics, and that beliefs about desire have been influenced by key advances (as well as key retreats) in science, feminism, psychology and sexology.

This first chapter is not intended to give a comprehensive and complete review of this history, as this would be an enormous feat, outside of my expertise and also, probably, not the reason you picked up this book. Nonetheless, these historical influences leave such a legacy it would be remiss of me not to mention how influential they still are for our sex lives today.

In this chapter I will give a brief, non-linear and selective historical overview in order to provide you with a foundation that will help you to make sense of later chapters and look at things you previously believed to be truths about sex with new eyes. I wish to demonstrate that how we view sex is almost entirely influenced by the prevailing culture, language and politics of the time, and attitudes to sex vary enormously across continents, communities and cultures because of this.

For the purpose of this book, I will focus on some of the key institutions that have dominated society in the UK as well as Western science over the last few centuries, which is not to say that there weren't other influences, or that there weren't other communities with different views and experiences at that time – there most definitely were. Dominant institutions and movements during this time, such as Christianity and monogamy, have had a tremendous impact on our views about sex and women's sexuality. Similarly, cultural shifts, such as the women's movement, had a significant impact on women's rights, sexuality and autonomy. And, in the twentieth century, the evolution of modern science and the birth of psychotherapy and sexology each played a significant and prevailing part in how society saw women and sex, all of which has laid the foundations for how we understand sex today.

To sum up, how we see sex, including what is 'normal' and how women are expected to relate to sex, is a moveable feast, depending on the cultural context and dominant views of the time. Although it may not seem like it, these key points in history are still hugely relevant to your sex life in this present moment.

Sex and sinning

We start this timeline in the seventeenth century, mainly because we have to start somewhere and the dawn of time would take us far too long. In many parts of the Western world, monogamy was the norm at that time, mainly due to the influence of religion and the importance given to the institution of marriage. Marriage had importance as it was connected to ownership of land and, therefore, finance, but most women's partners were chosen by their fathers, not by the women themselves. Christianity was the dominant influence on moral values, but the Protestant Reformation was gradually changing the image of marriage to something that was more about personal choice, and included desire, rather than almost exclusively being about procreation.[1] Interestingly, prior to this point in history, women had been considered to be the more lustful sex, but this was soon to change and be replaced by the idea that men's sexuality was more powerful and women were naturally less sexual. Sex outside of marriage and for anything other than procreation was seen as sinful, and this was evident in the laws of the time, with adultery and homosexuality being considered illegal and even punishable by death.

In contrast, it has been suggested that the eighteenth and nine-teenth centuries brought with them a shift in sexual values.[2] It was no longer illegal to have sex outside of a relationship (though still frowned upon), although women's sexuality was viewed as less powerful than men's, and women were positioned as 'gatekeepers' regarding sex, with the onus on men needing to control their urges. There was also an assumption that women's orgasms were important, as the woman's orgasm (and, in fact, a simultaneous orgasm) was believed to be crucial to getting pregnant. Sex was seen as an important part of marriage, but fears about the dangers of masturbation for one's physical and psychological health were prevalent. This was evident from the invention and dissemination of devices to prevent 'self-touch' and the lengths that people went to dampen sexual impulses, especially in women, for whom a percep-tion of a 'naturally' lower interest in sex meant that any evidence of sexuality was particularly problematic.

You could be forgiven for thinking that some of these more sex negative aspects of history were just representative of the times, represented across the world, and that we've moved on a lot since then. Not so. Many of these historical views of sex contrast greatly to more liberal attitudes to sex in the UK before this period, and also across the globe. Sex positivity is evident in numerous historical texts, such as the ancient Hindu *Kama Sutra* (compiled between 400 BCE and 200 CE) and the *Encyclopaedia of Pleasure* from tenth-century Baghdad.[3] In both of these, sex is represented as being primarily for pleasure, without shame and with relaxed attitudes to gender and sexual diversity. In many parts of the world it was, in fact, colonization by the British which imported more restrictive sexual values and brought with it new, more conservative perspectives. We also know that the sex = shame rhetoric is (and was) absent in many other non-Western cultures. Women living in certain matriarchal communities, such as those of the indigenous people of Papua New Guinea, were free to enjoy sexual expression with a variety of men for pleasure. What we can deduce from this is that, here in the UK and in other parts of the West, the roots of our recent sexual past are related to a conservative ancestry with views of sex related to religion, gender inequality, a fixation on monogamy, and with a distinct fear of sexual urges as the backdrop.

Sex and madness

Sex then moved from something that was policed by religion – 'your desires are a sin' – to something that was policed by medical science (at this time, psychiatry) – 'your desires are a sign of madness'. 'Hysteria' was defined as an illness connected to sexuality in women, with masturbation being one of the symptoms, while the term 'nymphomania', which was coined in the eighteenth century and rapidly gained popularity, was used to describe women who masturbated, wanted sex more than their husbands did, who fantasized about sex or who had sex with other women. The use of these terms as explanations for a range of women's experiences neatly aligned women's sexual urges with madness. Interestingly, at the turn of the nineteenth century, many more women were committed to psychiatric institutions than men for concerns regarding their sexual behaviour, a pattern and a narrative of female sexuality being seen as more dangerous than men's that we have not seen replicated since. Women were locked in psychiatric institutions, forced to have hysterectomies or lobotomies, had leeches applied to their genitals, were forced to take freezing cold baths, had their clitorises removed or caustic chemicals inserted into their vaginas. These diagnoses and treatments have been hypothesized to be a form of social control over women, with sexual desire as the mobilizing factor.

Sex and subjugation

In the second decade of the twentieth century, Britain was about to go to war. This devastating event marked a significant change in women's opportunities and position in society. Women were, for the first time, taking on roles that had typically been held by men in our historically patriarchal culture, shifting the view of what women were capable of. By the end of the Great War, significantly more women were in employment than had ever been before. Women, empowered by this experience, continued to push for rights that were justifiably theirs and, as a result of the efforts of the women's movement, some women were granted the right to vote in 1918. It has been suggested, however, that this small but significant shift in gender equality was met with a cultural backlash, as it was seen as potentially threatening to the institution of marriage, 'family values' and, therefore, society.

At the same time, modern science and medicine as we now know it was an evolving field, as was the means to carry out scientific enquiry. In the eighteenth and nineteenth centuries, a cultural shift from religion as a dominant world view to science as a dominant world view started to gain traction. This was not without challenge, as advocates of these two opposing views battled for who was right. A key feature of this era was that, until this time, it was dangerous to hold a view that represented something other than the dominant view of the church. Pretty soon, however, science became the more dominant voice (alongside religion and social convention) as an authority on people's lives, and this started to play out in sex, medicine and the control of women's sexuality by these means.

The creation of sexual dysfunctions

Psychiatry, it can be argued, created sexual dysfunction. The American Psychiatric Association's Diagnostic and Statistical Manual (DSM) was created in 1952, with the aim of being a complete list of all the possible diagnoses available regarding mental 'disorders'. Essentially, if it's not in there, it doesn't exist. But, equally, the inclusion of supposed disorders in DSM gives them credibility. The DSM first included sex as something which could be 'disordered' in the third edition, which came out in 1980.[4] Before this, people had concerns about sex, of course, but DSM-III marked the first time that specific terms for sexual problems (such as 'Inhibited sexual desire') were coined, a historical moment of which the aftermath influences our sex lives even now. Before this date, 'sexual dysfunctions' didn't have labels, weren't medicalized, and decisions about what aspects of sex to prioritize and therefore name 'dysfunctions' weren't decided upon on the basis of what constituted 'normal sex' at the time.

Sex and neuroses

In the late nineteenth and early twentieth centuries, a few determined voices started to suggest that religion and science had got it wrong when it came to sexual expression. Sexologists were few and far between, but those that were about, such as Havelock Ellis, were presenting very unpopular ideas, such as the thought that homo-sexuality was, in fact, not an illness but a normal representation of sexual preference found in humans.[5] Sex between men wasn't decrim-inalized until 1967 in the UK (and then not in all circumstances), however, and 'homosexuality' was only removed from DSM in 1973 (and so declassified as a 'mental disorder'). Sex between people of the same sex has been present in humanity since records began, and it hasn't always been seen as a problem by various cultures and communities through various points in history. And yet negative opinions about LGBTQ people are still painfully evident today when we look at the recent protests by parents in the UK against the inclusion of teaching around LGBT identities in schools.

When Sigmund Freud, the Austrian neurologist and psychiatrist, later dubbed the 'father of psychoanalysis', came along in the late nineteenth century, he was happy to talk about sex. So happy, in fact, that it seemed that everything was suddenly about sex in one way or another. Freud's own version of therapy came along before therapy began to utilize scientific methods, and his personal observations or reflections on his cases were postulated as theories that continued to dominate the world of psychotherapy for the next century. Much of Freud's theories about sex and sexuality we now know not to be true; for example, the idea that a clitoral orgasm is an 'immature' version of a vaginal orgasm, or that homosexuality is an immature version of heterosexuality. Despite unknowingly and unhelpfully pathologizing large sections of the population, at least Freud promoted a narrative about sex as something that people like to do, and an urge that people have, rather than the old narrative of sex being something to create life only (unless you're mad).

One of the most pivotal moments in sex science came with the ground-breaking work of Alfred Kinsey in the 1940s. Kinsey was an American entomologist (i.e. his field was the scientific study of insects) who decided to study human sexuality in a laboratory setting to learn more about it. Here we have the intersection of several key moments in time coming together in historical union. The view that sex is not a sin, but just something people do (and enjoy!) and also the view that everything can be observed and studied by science, just like you might study insects. And finally the concept that this is how we can come to know better what sex is or how people do it, not through opinion, the views of the church or the views of the state.

Through his interviews, Kinsey discovered that sexual orientation wasn't binary and that most people were somewhere in the middle, not on either end of a straight-or-gay scale. He discovered that people enjoyed sex, went about it in all sorts of different ways, and that most people masturbated. He suggested that all types of sexual expression were acceptable. Kinsey's work and discoveries were seen as so challenging to American family values that his funding was pulled, and his ground-breaking research was stopped in its tracks. If Freud was the father of psychotherapy, Kinsey was certainly the father of sexology.

Virginia Johnson and William Masters came next, and wanted to build on Kinsey's discoveries of what people do and find out more about how sex actually worked. Masters was a gynaecologist and Johnson was initially his research assistant and then became his partner – in both senses of the word. Throughout the 60s and

70s they applied science and process to their laboratory studies, making observations and collecting data on sex. Masters and Johnson came up with the first real model of what happens to humans during sex – the human sexual response cycle. This model was added to by Helen Singer Kaplan and others shortly after, and became *the* model to explain humans and sex for decades to come.[6]

The Masters and Johnson/Kaplan model (which you will learn more about in Chapter 7) not only formed the basis of all of the sexual dysfunctions that were first named in DSM and stayed there until very recently, but seeped into the fabric of society, from the echelons of science down to popular culture, and added to our idea of what sex is and how it should look. Masters and Johnson were quite keen on using the media to disseminate their discoveries to the masses and appeared regularly on TV, which was quite unusual for scientists of their time. I like to think of them as the original sex influencers and think that, if they were around right now, they'd have a massive Instagram following.

Masters and Johnson's understandings have formed the basis of how we as a society view 'normal' sex – even up until this day, and until now you may not have even realized that their work has been responsible for how *you* understand sex. This, of course, is what happens with science and law: if something is illegal, we presume it must be wrong, and if something is found in science, we presume it must be right. Without question we absorb these things to be truths and they form part of our cultural narrative. One of the key under-standings from Masters, Johnson and Kaplan was the idea that desire is the first part of human sexual response. These days, a large body of evidence suggests that this is not the case and that desire operates differently to how it was first understood in the 60s. This knowledge has not yet trickled down into mainstream understandings, but by the end of this book I hope you will have changed how you see desire completely, in line with these new views.

The potential for sex to be seen as a learnt skill is also perhaps a hangover from how sex was reported by the media around the time of the Masters and Johnson era, and an attitude which prevails even now. The question 'Are they good in bed?' suggests that we believe that sex is something we can be good at, as if having sex was like playing the piano or some other acquirable skill. In fact, sex is more like creating a piece of music and playing it in synchronicity with another musician, who has created their own piece, which yours must harmonize with. The skill is in listening and harmonizing, not simply playing the instrument.

Masters and Johnson are also credited with being the original founders of sex therapy, and so they should be. They published one of the first books on working with sexual problems and developed a new form of behavioural sex therapy. So much of their work is relevant now, and although sex science has moved on in leaps and bounds since then, their work still remains pivotal. What is fascinating about the work of Masters and Johnson is that, similar to Kinsey, their work also came at an important intersection in history.

At the time they were studying sex in the 1960s, behavioural and cognitive therapy paradigms were starting to take shape, and the dominant view of other models of therapy, descending from Freud, were making room for new ways of understanding how people think and how problems are formed. Much of Masters and Johnson's work was based on these behavioural and cognitive concepts. For example, they described how, if you have a thought that you will lose your erection, it causes anxiety in your body, which creates physical changes in the body, which in turn make sexual arousal (and therefore erections) impossible. The thought itself can cause the sexual problem, and the prediction of the same thing happening in the next sexual situation you find yourself in will mean that this cycle continues, building up momentum over time. These realisations were pivotal for sex therapy, as they moved us away from ideas of neuroses leading to sexual problems to the concept that sexual problems can happen to all of us, and can be overcome by creating a different experience or understanding. The continued influence of this approach will be evident as you read this book.

Sex and drugs – the medicalization of women and sex

Sex therapy as a field grew from the work of Masters and Johnson, gaining popularity, acceptability and kudos. But the advent of the pill in the 1960s brought with it a fresh panic about women's sexuality and what would happen to women's sexual behaviour without the restrictions of the fear of getting pregnant. Sadly, the ongoing policing of women's bodily autonomy is still a massive worldwide issue in relation to abortion rights, and there are strong parallels to be drawn around such restrictions and women's sexual lives in the world around us today.

In 1996, after the accidental discovery of Viagra by Pfizer, the field of sexology took a temporary medical diversion. Viagra had been designed to treat angina, but it was discovered that, as a side effect, it could produce rock-hard erections and drug companies immediately started to see pound signs (dollar signs, really, as it happened in the United States, but you know what I mean). There was suddenly much talk about creating a similar product for women. After all, it was 'well known' that women were not that keen on sex, compared to men, and that men supposedly needed more sex than women, so a fix to this problem seemed ideal (these things aren't actually true, of course, but bear with me). Drug companies raced to be the first to come up with a solution to the 'problem' of women's desire. In the background, a bunch of feminist scientists and sex therapists started to question the status quo about how women's sex lives (especially desire) were being talked about in the scientific and medical arena, with an absence of context about other forces that shaped women's sexuality.

Since 2015, two drugs have been approved by the Food and Drug Administration in the US for the treatment of low desire in women. The first was Flibanserin (Addyi) and, in 2019, Bremelanotide (Vyleesi). Both are associated with significant side effects reported in studies of their early use and there has been a great deal of controversy and debate about these drugs in the field of sexual medicine. Addyi brought a (rather unimpressive) increase of one extra satisfying sexual experience roughly every two months for the women taking it daily, with some challenging side effects and contraindications.[7] Controversy about such treatments is focused on the potential for further over-medicalizing women's sexual functioning and concern that situating women's desire in a purely medical context is reductive because it does not take into account the socio-political context women's relationships exist within. Despite the availability of Flibanserin and Bremelanotide in other parts of the world, medications specifically aimed at women with 'low desire' are not available in the UK currently, but this might change in the next decade, with several new drugs in development set to launch in Europe.

Sex, power and feminism

Until the 1960s, sex science (in fact, most science) was dominated by men, and we now know that this made a difference to the information that was gathered, the questions that were asked and the models that were put forward. Masters and Johnson studied sexual response in both men and women, and documented differences between the sexes – for example, making the discovery that women did not need the refractory period (the period of delay between orgasming and getting sexually aroused again that we see in men) and could be multi-orgasmic. But Masters and Johnson still landed on a final one-size-fits-all model of human sexual response that was predominantly based on a male experience (i.e. with a refractory period). This was a reflection of science as a patriarchal institution.

As such, we did not question whether the categories of sexual dysfunction that had been included in DSM since the 80s were perhaps better suited to heterosexual cis gendered male sexuality and maybe privileged penis-in-vagina sex over all else. Or that this bias didn't adequately represent anyone or anything else. For example, 'premature ejaculation' was defined in DSM-IV as 'coming before or just after vaginal penetration'. There was no equivalent category of coming too soon for women (even though we now know that a small proportion of women feel they do) or for coming too soon before another type of sex, such as mutual masturbation or anal penetration. The reason for this, as suggested by many sex scholars and academics, is that the only sexual dysfunctions included in DSM were ones which prevented the successful completion of wider society's current idea of what constitutes 'normal' sex, with men's experience taking centre stage. It doesn't matter when women come, as sex can continue, right? It also doesn't matter what happens for LGBTQ people, as straight cis sex is the *normal* one.

Feminist sex scientists and clinicians rejected these ideas of women's sexual difficulties based on this male model and patriarchal view of what sex is or who sex is for and formed a working group to address their concerns. In the early 2000s, 'The New View' of women's sexuality was proposed, as an alternative system for women, to move away from the perceived inequality and gender bias of DSM and the medical model.[8] This system allowed greater emphasis to be placed on the social, economic and political influences on women's sexuality. Leonore Tiefer, a vital member of this working party, used the analogy that 'sex is more like dancing than digestion', referencing the cultural, political, social and learned aspect of sex as more important than the historical importance placed on biology. You will see the influence of this view in this book, as I will talk very little about the biology of sex and desire, favouring instead the influence of society, gender politics, psychology and relationship dynamics.

Women started to play a more pivotal role in sex science and there was an explosion in the numbers of female sex researchers who, through their research and writing, have changed the way we see sex for ever. The work of many of them, such as Cynthia Graham, Rosemary Basson, Amy Muise, Sarah Murray, Robin Milhausen, Emily Impett, Lori Brotto, Meredith Chivers, Debbie Herbenick, Kristen Mark, Karen Blair, Caroline Pukall, Julia Heiman, Ellen Laan, Marta Meana, Sari Van Anders, Lisa Diamond and many equally important others, are represented in much of the scientific content referenced in this book. They have made discoveries and developed theories about sex and desire that will have a direct impact on how you understand your own. Remember their names, as they will go down in history, just as Kinsey or Masters and Johnson have, for the impact they have made to sex science. They are feminism, sex science and power in action.

In the last twenty years, perhaps the largest advances in sex science have been made with regards to how we understand women's desire. New models of sexual response were proposed to rival Masters and Johnsons, and, for the first time ever, they were based on women's sexuality, which I'll tell you more about in Part Two. Sex researchers started to learn more about women's desire, pleasure and orgasms and began to directly challenge the way women's sexual problems were represented in DSM, suggesting that, based on new science, the current classification system was pathologizing the normal expression of sexual functioning in women. New advances were made in understanding how attention and sex were closely linked, as well as the impact of our thoughts and how we experience relationships.

In the late 2000s, a team of sex scientists aimed to change the way women's desire was represented in DSM, based on new evidence, and they succeeded in creating a new category, 'Female sexual interest/arousal disorder', in the latest version of DSM, DSM-V.[9] The old category of Hypoactive (low) sexual desire disorder was removed, reflecting new research regarding how women find it hard to separate desire and arousal and placing much more emphasis on the subjective and relational aspects of arousal and desire. Such changes represent great strides forward in sex science, as opinions of what constitutes normal or dysfunctional in the scientific or medical community influences what we all believe of ourselves.

It is no longer seen as a problem if women don't feel like sex spontaneously. It is no longer seen as a problem if women don't feel like sex without 'adequate sexual stimuli' (for the record, for most people, saying 'It's been a while, how about a shag?' doesn't constitute 'adequate stimuli'). Women's sexuality, pleasure and capacity to respond to sex is being given the credit and attention it deserves, and the situations that amplify it, and extinguish it, are now understood in greater detail. Women are being armed with the information they need to know that their bodies work just fine.

2

Mind The Gap – Statistics around sex and desire

How much sex are people having?

I don't meet many people who *aren't* concerned about the amount of sex that they want or are having, or how their sex life is going more generally. You might feel that this is connected to the job that I do, but, in actual fact, this is what I hear both from my clients and the people I meet outside my job. Admittedly, once people find out what I do, they tend to share more with me about the details of their private life than they probably share with most. If we're ever at the same dinner party, I recommend sitting next to me, as inevitably the conversation in the immediate vicinity will turn to sex in some way, shape or form. The good thing about this for me is a) I love my job and never get tired of it, and b) sex is ridiculously fascinating and never gets boring, even when you talk about it all day.

People mainly start to worry because they are mapping out what's happening for them against a standard that they believe is the 'average'. But, generally speaking, people are drastically wrong when it comes to this estimation of other people's sex lives, and they are also often mistaken when it comes to the assumption that frequency is a good indicator of a good sex life (more on this later on). Still, I feel it's useful at this point to talk more about what's 'normal', so that you can feel reassured about what's happening for you. This is what this chapter is all about: a snapshot of our sex lives and what we know about what is *really* happening. A yardstick for you against which you can breathe a sigh of relief, but also an indicator of how inaccurately we understand and judge 'sex' as a society.

In this chapter I will lay out some of what we know from large-scale sex studies about how often people are having sex, the difficulties that we are having in our sex lives, and the consequences people report in relation to their lives and relationships generally when their sex lives aren't going to plan. I'll give you a sense of how common sexual dissatisfaction is and all the ways it can feel difficult, and (hopefully) begin to reassure you that, if you are struggling with these things, or would just like your sex life to be a bit better than it is now, it's not just about *you* or even your relationship, but rather something you share with a significant number of other women in the UK and the rest of the world.

Who decides what's normal?

One of the problems with sex is that, if you don't make the study or practice of working with it scientific, all you are really left with is bias, opinion, and the skewed impact of cultural values and assumptions. This is more the case with sex than it is with almost any other subject, as it is both something we don't talk about that often in public and (as we learned in the last chapter) it has been heavily dictated to by ideas of shame, religion, culture, medicine and politics at different points in history, giving a bias to which stories are privileged over others.

Not looking at sex scientifically (and by this I mean finding out what people do, and understanding how and why, by looking closely at the evidence rather than what you think) does not make for a good sex therapist. It also stops us learning more about sex as a society. As a clinical psychologist, the ethos of my training is about being an evidence-based practitioner. This means doing therapy based on what science says, not my intuition or assumptions. Of course, this doesn't mean I can't use my intuition at all, just that I should be careful to test my intuition as a hypothesis, rather than following it blindly. I use the learnings of science heavily in my therapy sessions, and my hope is that you will also value this aspect when reading this book.

It is for this reason that, the first time I heard about the Natsal study (National Survey of Sexual Attitudes and Lifestyles)[1] venturing into the realm of sexual functioning many years ago, I nearly fell off my seat in excitement. My joy was not just based on the fact that I knew it would provide us with solid facts about the sex life of the UK that we had never had on such a large scale before, but also because I'm a total sex-research geek. I feel we should be immensely proud of the fact that this study happens in our small country, especially as it is currently the biggest and most rigorous undertaking regarding sex research, on a population level, anywhere in the world. Natsal is a collaboration between several big research bodies and institutions and aims to look at how adults in the UK of all ages, backgrounds, ethnicities and sexual orientations experience sex, sexual health and, more recently, sexual function and satisfaction. It's one of the best markers we have about what *actually* happens in peoples sex lives, and without it we (as clinicians, but also as people having sexual relationships) are left completely in the dark about what's 'normal',* or how other people feel about or experience sex. Without this kind of research we are left only with societal opinions, based on skewed

---

* Although I've used the word 'normal' in this context, I do not mean that if you do something differently, or at a different frequency to the majority of the population, you are not 'normal'. Rather, there are things that are *common* sexually, and if these things happen to you or feature in your sex life, you can rest assured that you are not alone in this.

assumptions and biases, plus the dominant forces of the time in question, and you've already learned what a mess relying on that got us into historically in Chapter 1.

A national barometer of sex

One of the most crucial of the 'gaps' in our sex lives that the title of this book refers to lies between our perception of how our sex lives *should* be in comparison to others versus our lived experience of our actual sex lives. Frequency of sex is often a barometer that we use to judge this, possibly as it's easier to 'count' than some other aspects of sex. And, of course, we've been sold the myth that frequency is the most important thing (one of a whole host of myths, actually).

Over the last few decades, Natsal data tells us that the frequency that we're having sex has dropped in the UK, and a recent Natsal publication[2] tells us that, in the UK, the average person has sex a little less than once per week, or about three times per month (although this is more like twice a month for women between the ages of 35–44). This most recent analysis of the data also shows us that a higher proportion of adults under forty-four are reporting no sex at all in the last month, which is more than in previous Natsals (29% having no sex in the last month in Natsal 3, compared with 23% in Natsal 2).

This same Natsal publication also highlights general declines in sexual frequency in other countries around the world, such as Japan, Australia, Finland and the US, albeit showing slightly different trends in these declines. Now, firstly, don't panic if you're having sex a lot less than twice or three times a month, even if it's much less than this. What you will learn as we go on is that the frequency with which you have sex is almost meaningless. Do be reassured by these numbers, though, if you (or your partner) have been feeling abnormal based on your assumption that you should be having sex much more than this up until now. There's also nothing wrong with wanting more sex than you're having at the moment or more than is reported as the UK average. This Natsal data also picked up that over 50% of women (and even more men) wanted to be having *more* sex than they were currently having, but whether this is about people feeling their sexual frequency is not measuring up to a perceived norm, or whether people are genuinely dissatisfied with the amount of sex they are having we just don't know.

How frequently you want sex and how frequently you have sex are certainly not the same thing, and as we will learn over the course of this book, there any many factors that influence whether we invest in and act on our desires using the behaviour of 'sex'. Similarly, frequency of sex and quality of sex are not the same thing, and quality of sex has huge implications for desire. Often social chat about sex tends to be focused on *how much* sex people are having, or whether they *went all the way* (penetration), and very rarely how *mutually pleasurable* or even *life-expanding* it was. This is important, as alongside making people who have infrequent but life-affirming sex feel like their sex life isn't up to scratch, we know that frequent but unsatisfying sex is generally bad for desire and not actually a useful goal to aspire to anyway.

Sexual satisfaction and problems

Natsal was pioneered by a team of female scientists with expertise across public health, social science and epidemiology. It was conceived as a response to the beginning of the HIV epidemic in the UK in the late 1980s, when it became clear that the fight to combat HIV by reducing transmission would be impossible without a clear idea of the types of sex the population of the UK was having. The Natsal team have undertaken this enormous task every ten years since then, with data first coming out in 1990–91, then 1999–2001, and the latest in 2010–12. Natsal 4 is in the pipeline at the time of going to press. Over the years, Natsal's data gathering has intelligently evolved to include sexual function, as well as Sexually Transmitted Infections (STIs) and sexual behaviour.

Natsal 3 uncovered some key information about the sex lives of the UK, specifically that we have a high percentage of people reporting sexual problems.[3] Just over half of women (51%) and 42% of men reported a sexual problem, such as lack of interest in sex, lack of enjoyment in sex, difficulty reaching orgasm or erectile problems, lasting three months or more in the last year. Sexual problems were experienced across the age ranges. To put this into perspective, there were 15,000 adults surveyed across the country between the ages of 16–74, selected to represent a range of geographical locations and other demographics, and roughly half of these reported that something wasn't going as they felt it should in their sex life. This is an awfully large number, but does map on to similar studies done in the US, Australia and Europe (rates in non-Western countries are higher still), so it's both surprising and unsurprising in equal measure.

In Natsal 3, people were asked about how their body worked sexually, how they felt about their sex life, and how their sexual relationship was functioning. They found that difficulties with sex were associated with depression and poor physical health, relationship difficulties and finding it hard to talk about sex with a partner. When asked whether they had experienced sexual problems lasting three months or more in the past year, 34% of women in the UK reported a lack of interest in sex, 16% reported difficulties with orgasms, 13% an uncomfortably dry vagina and a further 12% reported a lack of enjoyment in sex.

This book is not focused on men's sexual experience, but you may also be surprised to hear that lack of interest in sex was the most commonly reported concern for men too, at just under 15%, quashing some ever-present myths that men are always wanting or ready for sex. Early ejaculation for men and anxiety during sex for women were two of the sexual concerns that decreased with age for men and women, reflecting perhaps the impact of growing sexual confidence over an individual's lifespan.

Consider these statistics for a second. Fifty-one percent of women reporting a sexual problem. A third of women feeling that they lacked interest in sex for a significant period of the previous year. This statistic is not surprising to me, as my clinic is full of women concerned about their desire, and feeling a lack of interest in sex is well known to be the most common reason that people seek sex therapy, but what do you make of this statistic? Consider your friendship group, your team at work or the people sitting around you on the bus / tube / train just now. Half of these women are dissatisfied with sex, and for just over 3 in 10 of them, this is connected to how much they feel like sex. This is where our sex lives are at in the UK. It's no wonder that drugs like Flibanserin have been developed, promising a 'quick solution' to this issue. And no wonder the therapy rooms of people like me are filled with couples desperate to fix this 'problem' in their relationship.

It's important to note, however, that there's a difference between having a sexual problem and feeling distressed by it. Of women reporting lack of interest in sex, pain or difficulty with orgasms, only 29% found their problem distressing.[4] This may tell us that a significant number of women with a sexual problem are coping with it okay, and don't interpret this issue around sexual functioning as a problem for them, or perhaps they have found a way around it.

The impact of sex on relationships

You might be wondering why it matters. I mean sex is just sex, right? A frivolous activity that we do in private for fun, not a life-or-death matter. Well, not exactly. Sex is more important to us as humans than we often give it credit for. In fact, research has found that people rate a happy sex life as more important than an adequate income or shared interests with a partner.[5] I would argue that part of the reason we don't give it credit for being as important as it is is that we don't understand the function it serves in our lives and relationships. But, for now, let's look at the evidence. What do we know about the impact of sexual dissatisfaction on peoples' lives? Does it make a difference to our overall happiness if our sex lives are going well?

Studies have shown that, when couples have sex, they are more likely to report a better mood and relationship satisfaction on that day and the next day or two afterwards.[6,7] In fact, there's evidence to suggest that sexual satisfaction might be more important to relationship satisfaction than relationship satisfaction is in having good sex.[8] I see this a great deal in my clinical practice. Yes, there is a link between relationship dissatisfaction and difficulties with sex[9] – it can obviously be difficult to have good sex if you are feeling angry, disconnected or disrespected by a partner. But I see many couples where it's the other way around. They describe a wonderful relationship, with sex the only part of it that is not working well for them. It may be that, for a while, they didn't mind this so much, and accepted that sex is the one part of their relationship that doesn't run as smoothly as the rest. But, over time, this became a concern for one or both of them, and they come to see me, wondering if it's possible for a great relationship and great sex to co-exist, or whether they need to accept that sex is the one area that isn't going to be so great. I've certainly worked with couples where all else in their relationship is good, but what's happening with sex has impacted on their relationship satisfaction or security over time.

The evidence is strong that having a good sex life is associated with relationship satisfaction and relationship stability,[10] and that maintaining desire has a positive effect on relationship satisfaction.[11] so, as much as we might like to think of sex as a frivolous recreational pursuit, there are some clear reasons why we might want to prioritize it if we want to maintain a happy relationship long term. There are numerous studies detailing the psychological and relationship consequences of an unhappy sex life. We know that, among other things, sexual problems are associated with decreased relationship quality, thoughts of infidelity[12] and lower personal well-being. When they have worries about their sexual desire, women typically describe a negative impact on their emotional health, self-esteem and their relationships,[13] with fears of consequences on the impact on their partner or relationship if it's not resolved.[14] Essentially, sex (when it's good) benefits our mood and is good for our sexual relationships all round. Not being happy with sex in a relationship can lead to resentment and feeling disconnected, or can leave one or both partners vulnerable to the idea of meeting their sexual needs elsewhere.

There are two obvious exceptions to this. The first is asexuality, a sexual orientation where you do not feel the need to have sex with another person. Asexuality is not the same as not feeling like sex much or only from time to time and being worried about it. People who identify as asexual feel no distress about their desire and their preferences about sex are fairly consistent over time (as with all sexual orientations, there can be some fluidity). A lack of sex in this case would not lead to the same personal or relational consequences, unless that person was in a relationship with someone who *did* wish to have sex and this caused a problem between them.

Secondly, these negative effects related to sexual dissatisfaction should not be extrapolated to situations of mutual agreed celibacy or consensual non-monogamy (CNM). In CNM relationships, one or both partners might have other sexual partners or sexual relationships, which might add to their overall sexual and relational happiness. In their 2016 paper,[15] Amy Muise and Emily Impett make the crucial point that 'no other relationship domain involves more dependence between partners than the domain of sexuality, given that the majority of long-term couples are monogamous and therefore cannot – or are not allowed to – get their sexual needs met outside of their current relationship'. They go on to discuss how, if there are other areas of relationship dissatisfaction, for example not feeling able to easily discuss work dilemmas with a partner, or not sharing the same interests, these needs can be met by others in our social or family circles, but not sex, if you are monogamous. It's important to note that consensual non-monogamy is a valid and healthy relationship structure, and allows people to make choices around sex and relationships which don't place all the responsibility upon one significant other to meet all an individual's needs. However, due to the social conventions and historical context I mentioned in Chapter 1, we often find ourselves being monogamous, without any real sense of having intentionally chosen it as the best fit for us; rather, we are monogamous by default, as it's *what people do*. It's worth considering this for yourself at this point. Did you choose to be monogamous as it feels like the best fit for you? Are there any drawbacks for you, such as those mentioned above? If you felt CNM was just as popular and it was celebrated by our society, would you be more likely to give it a try?

What are we distressed about?

Several research studies have demonstrated that women with sexual problems, such as concerns about low desire or difficulties with orgasm, feel more concerned about the impact of these issues on their partner than they do about the impact on themselves. This is particularly fascinating when you consider this in relation to the political context of gender equality that we discussed in Chapter 1. Why are we defining a good sex life based on someone else's satisfaction if we're not afforded the same concern in reverse?

We also know that women tend to worry more about a sexual difficulty the more 'severe' they think it is (as opposed to how severe it might objectively be)[16] and this, of course, is connected with what we think *should* be happening with our sex lives, which is especially relevant in the case of desire.

To sum up, we're concerned about the impact of how we are sexually, as it often doesn't match up to our ideas of what's 'normal' and we're concerned about the impact on a partner of how we are sexually more often than we are about the impact on ourselves.

How does desire change within a relationship over time?

How we feel in sexual relationships develops in different stages, beginning with a phase of infatuation and passion. This stage is characterized by the desire to be near each other constantly, lust, and obsessive thoughts. It is followed by a stage of greater emotional closeness and *companionate love*, where distance from the person is more easily tolerated. It's important to note that, typically, people experience higher levels of desire to have sex in the early stages of a relationship. After some time, when they enter more of a companionate love phase (roughly one to two years in), their levels of desire will typically reduce.[17]

It's extremely common for women to come to see me and blame this change in desire on themselves. Anna was a typical example, and described this as many other women have before her, saying 'It's fine at the beginning, I feel like sex a lot, but then, after some time, it just goes. It must be me that has the problem, as it happens in every long-term relationship I've been in.' If I had a pound for every woman who has consulted with me who compares her current sex life unfavourably with this unsustainable early sex life, and blames her faulty sex drive for it, I'd be quite well off. Wouldn't it be great if we knew that this was normal, rather than a problem with us or our relationships?

There are two important things to consider about this pattern of a change over time. The first is that, although a drop in desire from the first few months or year is common for many couples, it is certainly not the case that this drop in desire should lead to sexual or relationship dissatisfaction. The second is that desire declining over the course of a relationship doesn't happen for everyone,[18] and even though it's associated with the length of the relationship, this does not mean that time is the key factor which causes the decline. In fact, there are many other relational factors which might pick up speed over the duration of a relationship, such as predictability, equity/division of labour, amount of time spent connecting, the impact of having children, and too much or too little intimacy, all of which are more likely culprits. You'll be hearing all about these in Chapter 5, and the good news is that these are all areas you can nurture and create positive change in, should you wish to. It's likely that the couples who maintain desire over time are the ones who either know how, or instinctively nurture, these aspects of their relationship, and you can do the same. There is an important distinction here between knowing what's normal but at the same time not believing that this change should result in a worse sex life and an inevitable decline, so that we just give up aspiring to great sex. A decline in sexual satisfaction in a long-term relationship is not a given.

It's useful to note at this stage that physical attraction is important to desire,[19] and that there is research to suggest that being more physically attracted to a partner at the start of a relationship is a protective factor for desire later down the line.[20] However, I would also like to point out that changes in relationship dynamics can lead to a change in attraction (in either direction) as can a re-emergence of seeing each other as sexual beings again, both of which we will cover in Chapter 5. In my sex therapy work I notice that it can be hard for people to evaluate whether they still feel attracted to their partner when sex isn't going as well as they'd like, and it's not necessarily the case that they are not attracted to their partner, rather that they have stopped looking at their partner *in that way*. In my experience it can be useful to revisit the question of attraction again later on, when changes are in place which have shifted the sexual relationship to new territory.

It's also to be expected that our sex lives and desire will face challenges over time, and that this happens at different rates for each partner, so that there will frequently be times of mismatch that will need to be negotiated. Natsal 3's data showed that differences in sexual desire within couples are common, with about 1 in 4 people reporting a difference in their want for sex and their partner's, and other researchers have suggested that desire discrepancy should be thought of as inevitable in the context of a sexual relationship.[21] Similarly, what people desire will change over the course of a relationship too, and it's common for couples to have to navigate differences in the things they like sexually, and how often they do them. The key thing here is that having a good sex life is not about always needing to be on the same page, or wanting as much sex as your partner, but the success with which you navigate these differences.

Men are not from Mars

We have long believed that men want more sex than women. This is not consistently backed up by research, as it depends on how desire is measured, and we are starting to see more similarities than differences between men and women when we measure certain types of desire.[22] Also, expectations that we have for men, women and desire are learnt by the process of absorbing societal messages. Therefore, when men do report higher levels of desire than women, it's likely that this is, in part, related to the expression of gendered norms that they should, in the same way that women are socialized not to express high desire. Men are negatively impacted by the expectation that they should spontaneously feel like sex often, and that they should always be up for sex. Plenty of men have concerns that they don't feel like sex enough (if you remember, Natsal data reported it was just under 15%). The truth is that the force is strong when it comes to gendered expectations of behaviour for men and women and we are not as different as we are led to believe in many ways. Yes, androgens such as testosterone play an important role in sexual desire, and, yes, men generally have higher levels of androgens than women (though there's not as big a difference as you might think, and men and women show considerable overlap). But there is no clear difference in the levels of testosterone in women with high and low desire,[23] so we can't just look to hormones as the reason. As you will learn later on, although desire is dependent on biological processes in part, it is largely a psychological event underpinned by physical factors, not the other way around.

The other important factor, while we're on the subject of gender, is that gender is a social construct, and the key aspects of how biological sex and gender manifest in humans (such as hormones, neuroscience, chromosomes, genitalia and the social expression of gender) do not always show clear indications of a distinct gender binary (for example, in the case of people who are intersex).[24] This means that clear distinctions of the categories of 'male' and 'female' cannot be easily observed in science. As hard as it can be to get your head around this, our social categories of 'men' and 'women' are more of a convenient societal shorthand than a scientific fact. This means that there's plenty of variation between people who consider themselves to be male and female and therefore much crossover when it comes to the expression of sex and desire on many levels. One of the problems, though, is that our social convention of using binary gender is so entrenched that most research about sex is done with 'men' or 'women', hence my having to talk in this book as though gender is more binary than we now know that it is.

One of the interesting differences between desire in long-term relationships over time for men and women is connected to the length of the relationship, as mentioned earlier. Women's desire is more likely to decline for the same partner whereas men are more likely to maintain a sense of desire for the same partner over many years.[25] The challenge of the demands of monogamy for women has been written about eloquently by Wednesday Martin.[26] Martin brings together data from anthropology, history and sex science to understand female desire as not naturally monogamous and constrained in Western culture by the socio-political climate women find themselves in. The concept of long-term sexual exclusivity dampening female sexual desire has been researched and written about by others too, and it's certainly the case that the struggle many women have in maintaining desire in long-term monogamous relationships is accepted in sex science.

Another interesting fact about sexual satisfaction and gender from The Global Survey of Attitudes and Behaviours in 2005[27] is that differences in sexual satisfaction between men and women are more significant in countries with less gender equality, highlighting the important notion of women's political and social context being taken into account when it comes to sex, as proposed by The New View Campaign. It's perhaps an obvious thing to say, but without safety, agency, autonomy and equality of pleasure, women's desire suffers.

What's the right amount of desire?

I mentioned earlier that frequency of sex is not the same as frequency of desire. People often have sex when they don't feel like it, and don't get to have sex sometimes when they do. So, what do we know from research about how often women report feeling like sex? Studies have found that, when asked about their levels of sexual desire, a large proportion of women commonly say something between 'never' or 'once or twice a month'.[28] Studies such as these are vital in understanding that it is normal for many women to not feel like sex often out of the blue, and data such as this has also underpinned some of the new understandings of women's sexual desire in long-term relationships that you will learn about later on in this book.

But here's a fascinating fact: there are several conceptual problems with how we measure desire, which make it difficult for us to know for sure what is 'normal'.[29] The first is that we have moved away from an understanding of sex as a drive – something that we all have within us that is a fixed part of who we are. Now we understand that our desire is never static, and we have to remember that we are only really measuring desire in that exact moment. The second is that our new understandings of desire tell us that it is dependent on context, and so, when we ask about it, we are not learning about the levels of desire *within that person* but their current desire in that exact moment in *that particular context*. Their desire might show itself differently the week after, if their circumstances change. The third problem is that women's desire is now known to work best when triggered, rather than just occurring out of the blue, and therefore many of the old studies of gendered differences in desire asking 'how often do you think about/feel like/initiate sex?' were measuring the 'wrong type' of desire for women. With this new understanding, it's hard to measure women's desire without triggering it first. This means that a large proportion of women might say that they think about or feel like sex never, or once or twice a month, but if you transported these same women to a remote paradise, removed their daily stress and orchestrated an intimate and flirtatious week with a very touchy-feely Idris Elba, they might report thinking about and desiring sex several times a day . . .

So, despite us knowing that, when asked, women report never or rarely thinking about sex, there is no norm in sexual medicine for what our levels of sexual desire should be. Amazing, right? Where else in science is there no norm? We have norms for height, norms for intelligence, norms for how long it takes men to come etc, etc. These can all easily be displayed on a bell-shaped curve with an average in the middle and a range that we expect most people to fall within. Not desire. It's impossible to give a definitive, as the variance is too wide even within individuals, and desire is too situation specific. Desire is too dependent on everything else that is going on, in essence. It has the potential to vary significantly person to person, relationship to relationship, day to day.

In the much-improved definition of Female Sexual Interest/Arousal disorder, which replaced Hypoactive (low) Desire in DSM-V, as mentioned earlier, there are no criteria for frequency of desire for this very reason. Also, it is suggested that sexual interest should be assessed as a response to 'adequate triggers' to desire. One of the criteria for FSIAD is being distressed about it, which is important, as who cares if you have no interest in sex if you don't? Plus, this also usefully avoids asexual people being pathologized. This change to the diagnostic criteria is important. But there's a bit of a Catch-22 still in how we view desire until we as a society understand desire more thoroughly. We are upset that our desire isn't 'normal' (in the absence of there being a known normal), and we're likely basing this idea of normal on an unrealistic belief of spontaneous desire (we don't yet talk much about 'adequate triggers' or responsive desire when talking in our society, about 'low sex drive'). So, in some ways, we can meet the criteria of distress, at least, by not really knowing how desire operates.

My perspective is that, until popular culture catches up with the scientific understanding of how women's desire works, and how we might expect to feel, how women report their desire and the distress women experience in relation to it is entirely driven by unrealistic expectations, not necessarily a problem with their desire itself. This was one of the motivators for me to write this book, as I believe that helping women to understand how their desire works, what they can expect of it, and how to maintain desire in their relationships, could make a difference to the large numbers of women who are concerned that their desire isn't working the way it should.

There are two things I want you to take away from this chapter. The first is that the sexual life of the UK, on paper at least, would not pass its own MOT and there are huge potential psychological- and relationship-level consequences for such widespread levels of dissatisfaction and concern. The second is that these difficulties are so common and happen on such a widespread level that they are more likely a problem of how we understand and think about sex as a society rather than a problem with us or our relationships. We might think of the problem more as how we think of and understand sex, and the gap between how we expect our sex lives to be/work and how they actually are. The rest of this book is designed to help you spot how, as a society, we've got ourselves into this position, and crucially, how we can get ourselves out of it.

3

Gaps in our foundations

Gaps in our knowledge

Unless your sex education was startlingly different to mine, the key features of it were probably something like this: don't get pregnant, don't get an STI, and, actually, try not to have sex at all, okay?. Even better, if you went to a very religious school, like I did, you probably took away some other unhelpful nuggets, such as 'abortion makes you a bad person' and 'contraception is a sin'. Good luck navigating a straightforward road to sexual pleasure with those foundations.

Essentially, for many of us our early sex education was a mish-mash of scaremongering, finger-pointing and threats of impending disaster. Not only was there very little *sex positive* talk, of the myriad good outcomes that might come from sex, but for many of us there was also very little *sex neutral* talk, of sex being okay, really, all things considered. *Sex negativity* was the name of the game, and this message may have been amplified by the absence of talk about sex at home too. TVs switched over or slightly awkward faces, say, and not even the slightest hint of information about sex from our parents. For lots of us, this unhelpful experience has scarred our sexual lives from the get go, as we embarked upon our journey far too focused on avoiding all that could go wrong, and without the slightest regard for how it could go right. For girls and women especially, some of the first things we learned about sex were 'it's dangerous', 'you shouldn't really be doing it', 'nice girls don't', and 'you'll get yourself a reputation.' If you didn't identify as straight as a teenager or young adult, you will have had the added bonus of 'you and your sexual thoughts are not normal'.

The way we learn about sex shapes our perception of it. Many women are still psychologically imprisoned by the way in which the concept of sex was presented to them, as something shameful, dirty and not to be celebrated. We were programmed to pay attention during sex to all that can go wrong, not the things that can go right. There was a total disregard for our pleasure, as a barometer of how good it was: instead we were encouraged to look for signs that 'nothing went wrong' and 'they thought I was okay' as an indication that it qualified as 'good sex'. You will see in Part Two how much this early learning has disseminated throughout society, our relationships and our minds, to influence our sex lives in the here and now. This is something I will be encouraging you to move away from as a key part of navigating your way to your best sexual life.

Perhaps you had a slightly different experience than this and sex was talked about freely and easily in your house, bodies were celebrated and your parents happily took you to get the pill once you talked about being sexually active? I do hope this was the case. Research has demonstrated that young people who are more 'sexually competent' tend to have more positive sexual experiences and delay their first sexual experience. Crucially, early positive experiences in relation to sex education are associated with better sex lives later on.[1] 'Sexual competence' is a term that was first put forward in a paper by Kaye Wellings and team in 2001, in order to move away from the idea of age as an appropriate marker of readiness for first sexual experience, given that age is both arbitrary (two sixteen-year-olds can be quite different) and the societal definitions of the age of consent are based on opinion and have changed over time.[2] Wellings and her colleagues proposed that it might be useful to move away from definitions and studies of 'early sex' based on age alone and move towards definitions of timings of sexual debut that were more aligned with holistic concepts of sexual health and wellbeing. For this reason, they defined 'sexual competence' as making decisions to have sex which are autonomous (i.e. because you want to rather than as a result of peer pressure), where there is mutual consent, where the time felt 'right' and where there is adequate protection from STIs and unwanted pregnancy.

How sex positive was your sex ed?

We now know that it's not just sex neutral messages that we should be aspiring to as a society and as parents or carers of young people, but messages that are more clearly sex positive. It's great not to have any strong negative reactions to a young person telling you that they are sexually active, and to help them think through their options with regards to their sexual health; heck, it's better than the sex negative experience that many of us had. But it is even better to have frank and open conversations about celebrating pleasure, celebrating sex, and how we can work with our bodies and relationships to get the best out of them. Imagine for a minute what your relationship to sex now might have been like had you had a different introduction to it as a child/teen? If you were told about masturbation being a great thing, about sex being something wonderful when the time feels right, about the role of the clitoris in your pleasure, about the importance of respect and consent? If the focus had been about sex being something wonderful for you to look forward to, rather than something dangerous or morally wrong?

Many of us are working hard to reverse the damage that this sex negativity has done to our sex lives. We can choose to reject these sex negative ideas as adults, and to move towards representations of ourselves as sexual, as not only entitled to good sex but with the belief that it is good for us and our lives. We might need to surround ourselves with sex positive messages to do this, or to be able to notice the sex negative thoughts and reactions creeping in automatically and choose to reject them. But it *is* possible and, later on, I'll be telling you how. We also have a huge opportunity in front of us, as many of us are parents, caregivers, significant family members or role models for young people, and so we have a chance to change this for the next generation. As we learned in the last chapter, the benefits of good sex for people's life and relationship satisfaction is without question, but good sex can be harder to come by easily when there is a foundation of sex negativity. If you have any influence or contribution to the sex education of a child or young person, I urge you to consider the impact that the following might have on their sex lives as adults:

- Knowing the right words for their genitals and saying them without shame from as early as possible

- Knowing that (and how) their bodies can give pleasure and that this is wonderful

- Having a sense that their body is theirs, and they can do with it what they please, including saying no to others (i.e. not being forced to give Uncle Bob a hug just because he wants one)

- Understanding that variety in sexual and gender expression are perfectly okay and not presuming their gender identity as cis (aligned with their sex assigned at birth) or their sexuality as 'straight'

- Knowing what sex is, what it isn't, and what can be amazing about it (but not suggesting that sex has to be all about love or commitment)

○ Understanding the difference between porn and real-life sex

○ Understanding the choices available to them about avoiding pregnancy and STIs, but also that, once this is taken care of, sex does not need to be something to fear

It's important that good sex and relationship education happens in schools, of course, and we have made great strides with this in the last year alone in the UK. But I'm a firm believer that the responsibility belongs to parents and caregivers too, not solely with schools. This is because good sex education is a lifelong pursuit, and is just as much taught in attitudes to bodies, gender, consent and boundaries from early childhood as it is with talk of porn and contraception later on. It's something that is best done in a holistic, consistent and meaningful way by modelling and continuous conversation. There are some exceptional social media/web sites, such as the 'sex positive families' Instagram feed and website,* which provide guidance and resources to help parents and caregivers who didn't have this kind of education themselves, who struggle to know what it acceptable, how to do it and what to cover. If it's something you want to learn more about, do look into it and think of the impact that you could be having on a young peron's future sex and relationship satisfaction by laying solid foundations of sex positivity.

Anatomy and pleasure

For women (as well as trans and non-binary people with clitorises), the clitoris is really the source of our sexual pleasure; it contains

* https://sexpositivefamilies.com/

corresponding structures and nerve pathways to the penis. It's often not a part of our anatomy that we are particularly familiar with, or learn about when we are younger and are taught about at school, so it can come as a bit of a surprise to know that the tip of the clitoris (the glans, which is the pea-sized bit of it you can often see under the clitoral hood) is just the tip of the iceberg when it comes to its full function and structure. In fact, the clitoris extends about 9cm in length and 6cm in width underneath the skin, and the full structure looks a bit like this:

FULL STRUCTURE OF THE CLITORIS

Clitoral glans

Urethral opening

Bulb of vestibule

Crus of clitoris

Vaginal opening

The clitoris is equivalent in structure and function for pleasure to the penis, in that it fills with blood on arousal, and it is a key source of sexual pleasure when stimulated. Its sole job is to give pleasure.

Many people find it shocking that the full structure of the clitoris was only supposedly discovered and publicised in 2005, after we had already discovered life-saving HIV medications and had identified and mapped all of the genes of the human genome, but the real disappointment is that the full structure of the clitoris was actually first discovered in 1844, by the German anatomist Georg Ludwig Kobel; it's just that the scientific community decided not to include this discovery in most anatomical diagrams, anatomy texts or models of the female pelvis for the following century and a half. Mark Bletchner wrote a great paper about this, and how it's possible that the clitoris has been repeatedly discovered and then forgotten about again over the course of more than a century.[3] He also talks about the fact that it's perhaps no coincidence that most anatomists were men, a point which corresponds with our discussion of male bias in sex science from Chapter 1.

The full structure of the clitoris, however, resurfaced again in 2005, after surgeon Helen O. Connell and her team presented an MRI view of it[4] and it's received a fair amount more airtime since then, with people producing 3D models, jewellery, art, animations and fancy-dress costumes (brilliant!), but it's still often a surprise for many women and their partners to see it. Given the power for pleasure that the clitoris has, it's an enormous travesty that it is so often left out of discussions about women's genital anatomy in favour of other parts of our anatomy, such as the vagina, the uterus and the ovaries. Talk about women's sexual anatomy essentially privileges the parts that can make the woman useful to someone else and those that are problematized. The foundations of our knowledge are all wrong.

Perhaps if we talked about masturbation more we might feel more confident in understanding the clitoris in all its glory, and the key role that it must play in sex if we want pleasure to feature? For example, we know that most women who masturbate do so by stimulating the clitoris (with fingers, sex toys, an object) and that this is the most reliable route to orgasm for most, as it stimulates the glans of the clitoris directly, as well as the other internal structures behind it. It's common, also, for a smaller proportion of women to use vaginal penetration as an adjunct to this, to enjoy a different sensation, and given that the bulbs and legs (called crura) of the clitoris are either side of the vaginal walls, this sensation is also stimulating the clitoris, albeit less directly. What is uncommon is women using penetration as the sole act of masturbation, with no additional clitoral stimulation (it happens, but in less than 5% of women[5]). The statistics about what women do sexually when left to their own devices speaks volumes about what women's bodies need and respond to.

The orgasm gap

Nowhere are the gaps in the foundations of gender inequality and its impact on the sex lives of women more evident than in the orgasm gap between men and women when they have sex together. If you haven't heard of the orgasm gap already, it's basically the sex equivalent to when we found out that the BBC were paying men more than women to be on the same show. The orgasm gap situates the disadvantaged sex lives of heterosexual women as a feminist issue. It references several pieces of key research published in the last two decades, which tell us that:

○ Despite what we've been led to believe, women's bodies are *not* 'trickier' than men's. Women and men can orgasm at roughly the same rate from masturbation (over 95% of men and women can reliably orgasm this way in just a few minutes[6])

- When women and men have sex with each other, the rate of men usually or always orgasming stays at 95%, and for women it drops to 65%,[7] with much lower rates reported by women for casual sex (only a depressing 18% of women usually or often orgasming during casual sex[8])

- Women who have sex with other women do not see such a significant drop in orgasms when they have sex with each other (orgasm rates of 85%)

- The rates of how often woman have orgasms alone or with other women tell us that women have a similar orgasmic capacity as men

- From this we can deduce that it's not women's sexuality, capacity for pleasure or anatomy that is responsible for women coming less than men when women and men have sex together, but, rather, how sex happens and whose pleasure is prioritized

To make sense of the orgasm gap, we need to understand which types of sex are most associated with sexual pleasure and orgasm for women and how these fit with the types of sex that heterosexual women usually have.

I mentioned that the number one sexual activity for reaching orgasm is masturbation. Although a small proportion of women struggle to orgasm alone, most women reliably orgasm from masturbation even if they don't orgasm from other types of sex. Following masturbation, the second[9] is a partner using their hands to stimulate the clitoris, the third receiving oral sex and, lastly (very faint drum roll), penetrative vaginal sex.[10]

What's interesting is that, for heterosexual men, the activities resulting in 'usually or always' experiencing orgasm follow a different order. Penetrative sex is high up on the list, alongside masturbation, and, on average, men prefer penetrative sex to any other sexual act, such as receiving oral sex or manual stimulation by a partner's hand.[11] Despite this gendered difference in pleasure resulting from penetrative sex, it features much more highly in the sexual scripts of heterosexual sex than in same-sex experiences,[12] occurring at a much more frequent rate when men and women have sex together. One of the key differences in the sex lives of women who have sex with women is that they typically report a greater variety and frequency of sexual acts, such as receiving oral sex and clitoral stimulation, alongside penetrative sex. This shows itself in more orgasms (as well as more general sexual satisfaction) than women who have sex with men. Women who have sex together are also three times as likely as heterosexual women to have an orgasm with a partner, along with a greater frequency of multiple orgasms.[13]

Women's drop in orgasm frequency when having sex with men is a result of the type of sex men and women most frequently have together, not a result of women's ability to orgasm, but what's disheartening about this is that we know that women who have fewer orgasms tend to blame themselves rather than external factors, such as the types of sex they are having, or societal influences, for not coming.[14] But why? Well, it's the influence of society on what we believe to be 'normal' and how this plays out in the sexual scripts we feel we should enact.

'Sexual scripts' are pre-conceived, societally dictated norms about how we should behave during sex and, amongst other unhelpful ideas, lead us to believe that women's orgasms are elusive and should not be expected, that men's sexual pleasure is more important (especially when it comes to casual sex), and that the type of sex which equates to 'real sex' is vaginal penetration (suiting men's anatomy and their most reliable route to orgasm, not women's).

Although it's certainly the case that not all people know the significance of the clitoris for female sexual pleasure, or the fact that orgasms from vaginal penetration alone are rare for women, when women do know this information, it's associated with higher rates of orgasm from masturbation, yet does not translate into sex with a male partner.[15] So there's more to the orgasm gap than a lack of knowledge regarding what women like sexually; there's a whole host of other pressures, not to be 'too assertive', not to put our pleasure first if it impacts on someone else's, not to go against what we believe it expected of us sexually. We'll be revisiting sexual scripts and their influence on us in Chapter 4, but the acceptance of both the orgasm gap and men's pleasure taking precedence in heterosexual sex are certainly a stark indicator of patriarchy in action.

But it's also important to say that, if we remove the gender inequality of women not coming at the same rate as men, orgasms are not the be all and end all of good sex. There's plenty of other emotional, relational and physical rewards that sex can bring that we should be aiming for as part of our sexual experiences. Yet research tells us that women report more satisfaction with their sex life and relationships more generally when they have more orgasms,[16] so while we shouldn't see orgasms as the only goal of sex, we certainly shouldn't discount their role in overall sexual satisfaction either – especially when there is such a sizeable gap between men and women and the impact that sexual pleasure has on desire.

'Change me, not my sex life'

In my clinical work, I often have women come to see me because they are concerned about not being able to have orgasms. Once we get talking and I find out more, it's not unusual to find out that they do, in fact, have orgasms, just not from penetrative vaginal sex. They explain that they can orgasm from masturbation, and/or from receiving oral sex from a partner, for example, but that this doesn't feel good enough for them or their partner. Sometimes they are at first shocked, then usually reassured, to hear that this is normal for women and that most women can't come from vaginal penetration. In fact, the majority of women are not able to come from vaginal stimulation without any additional direct or indirect stimulation of the clitoris.[17]

Frequently women accept this, but then ask me how I can help them change this so that they can start having orgasms from vaginal sex. I explain to them that expecting a woman to orgasm from no stimulation to the clitoris is equivalent to expecting a man to orgasm from sex that includes no touch or stimulation to his penis. I sometimes ask them how open to that idea they think most men would be? They might laugh a bit at this point at the ridiculousness of the question, but underlying this is an important political point about women's sexual pleasure. As a society we still do not see women's sexual pleasure as being as worthy as men's. We are happy to achieve it, but only if the route to achieving it doesn't disrupt the experience for someone else ('someone else' usually being male, as women having sex with women are not as focused on this idea of having to change their body to create vaginal orgasms, in my experience). In 2020, women are still coming to people like me to find a way to circumvent their own anatomical needs to prioritize a man's.

The Orgasm Olympics

As a psychologist who works with people to help them get the sex life that they want, I'm totally uninterested in the current media focus on striving to achieve an almost tick-box-like holy grail of women's pleasure, as per articles such as 'The 14 Different Types of Orgasm', or 'The Quest for Female Ejaculation'. Sex is not a competition in which your body needs to be trained to do more and more. Pleasure is pleasure, orgasms are orgasms, and who cares how each of us get there as long as we have the knowledge about ourselves *to* get there. When it comes to sexual satisfaction, pressure on having to come in different ways or learn how to enjoy 'G spot' stimulation are missing the point entirely. Yes, explore your body in any way you like, and learn new things about yourself as you do it. That is certainly important. But good sex is about so much more than a technique, is so much more than a physical act. For this reason, you will see no 'how to' guides in this book, as tips, tricks and titillating techniques miss the point of what really matters: how you relate to your body, your gender, your relationship and yourself sexually, and how this helps or hinders how sex unfolds for you. It's these things that make sex worthwhile and sexual desire and satisfaction long-lasting.

Gaps in our language

The other problem we have with the foundations of our sexual understanding is the inaccuracy of language that we use to describe women's genitals. We are not only raised with huge gaps in our vocabulary in relation to our genitals but also with an absence of awareness that some parts of our body exist or what they exist for. A recent campaign by the Eve appeal, as part of their Gynaecological Cancer Awareness Month, revealed that 44% of women were unable to identify their vagina on an anatomical diagram, and 60% were unable to identify a vulva. My guess is that this percentage is significantly higher when it comes to the full anatomy of the clitoris.

For decades we've been using the word 'vagina' when we actually mean 'vulva', incorrectly locating the important parts of women's sexual anatomy in completely the wrong place. The widespread use of the word vagina suggests that the vagina (the canal leading up to the cervix and uterus) is what sex is all about for women, an inaccurate use of language which has reinforced untrue ideas of what women prefer sexually.

I feel passionately that there would be a huge shift in sexual satisfaction if we could just get this right. Knowledge is a crucial basis for our sexual satisfaction learning journey, and it helps us to navigate creating a foundation with someone else within which sexual satisfaction can thrive.

What is sex?

An important gap in the foundations of our knowledge about sex is what we actually see sex as being in the first place. My guess is that, if we asked 100 people on the street what 'sex' is, they would describe it as a physical act. Sex is, of course, physical, as it's often (but not always!) about something we are *doing* with our bodies, and the sensations this produces. Less often do people think of sex as psychological, i.e. about what's going on in our minds, or relational – how we are connecting with another person. Even more rare, I imagine, would be the proportion of this 100 people who would guess that sex is something we do that is an enactment of society/ culture. The truth is, it is all of these things. Sex is widely known in sex science to be a biopsychosocial phenomenon. What this means is that you can't separate what goes on in your body from what goes on in your head or from the relationship between you, other people and society. The crucial consequence of this in regards to having a 'good' sex life long term, especially when it comes to maintaining desire, is that each of these aspects are essential to the picture. Another reason why learning to 'orgasm from having your feet touched' is not going to salvage your sex life or protect desire from dwindling.

Understanding what makes sex good for us

Part of knowing yourself sexually and getting the most out of your sexual experiences is understanding what I call your 'conditions for good sex'. You can think of these conditions as an inter-related triangle, of which all three points are crucial to your sexual experience.

The three points of the triangle are:

Psychological arousal – this refers to how much of what is happening involves experiences or contexts that you find erotic, and how much the connection you have with that person meets these needs also. It involves things like the environment, trust, safety, love, power play, how exciting you find different sexual acts, visual stimuli, the dynamic or connection between you and your partner, talking, attraction, passion, props, sensuality, close-ness, eye contact, the role you take and much more. This part of the triangle can be thought of as how close this sexual situation matches up to the kind of sexual situation you would create in a fantasy, for example, or which would create maximum arousal.

Physical touch – this refers to how close the physical stimulation is to the type of physical stimulation that makes your body feel good. This can be anything from the type of kiss that you like to whether you like penetration or not (and if so, where), the pressure of touch you like to your skin, and the speed and location of touch to your genitals. It could be around restraint, fabrics, the feel of body hair, the feel of someone's body. There is some overlap here with the psychological, as a sexual position you enjoy could be both about physical touch (you feel the most pleasure in that position due to the contact between your bodies) but also psychologically arousing (as you find that position hot).

How present you are – this refers to how 'in the moment' you are, versus being away with your own thoughts or distractions. This can be anything from feeling worried, self-conscious and anxious, to being distracted by something innocuous in the background. There is a continuum here, with being totally in the moment or totally present at one end and being totally distracted by what's going on in your mind at the other. The reality is that we might be somewhere between those two points, but the closer we are to being present, the better.

In a 2007 paper investigating the key components of great sex, the authors Klienplatz and Menard state 'this quality of being entirely alive in their bodies with no mental interference was the hallmark of great sex'. Participants in the study described being present as 'Reaching the point where arousal overcomes thinking', and 'I stop the running commentary in my head . . . I don't have to think about where to place my hand – it just goes there.'[18] The opposite of this, of course, is a constant running commentary in your mind during the encounter, covering everything from 'Oh no, they will see that I've not shaved my legs!' to 'I don't think I'm ever going to come . . . should I tell them?' to 'Is that next door's cat I can hear?'

We want each of these three factors to be as close to our ideal conditions as they can be, so maximum eroticism through high levels of psychological arousal, the most pleasurable physical touch based on what we like, and being as present as we can be. The content of each of these three aspects will be different for all of us, and it's this reason that it's impossible to be 'good at' sex, as you can never really know what someone else's conditions will be without asking or being told. In this case, you might be good at talking about sex, or responding to feedback – both of which are great skills for sex, as we will learn later – but the phrase 'good at sex' is a societal term which implies that there is a 'right' way to do sex that works for most people, and this is simply not the case.

If we feel really turned on (high psychological arousal), are receiving pleasurable physical touch and have a low level of distraction or worry, we are meeting our 'conditions for good sex' and it's more likely that this sex will be pleasurable for us. Our 'conditions for good sex' do not exist in isolation, of course, and there are additional external contexts which impact upon it, such as understanding what needs sex is meeting for us at any given time, negotiating and communicating what we want with someone else, and how much our conditions feel accepted or frowned upon by society. These further aspects will all be explored later on in this book. However, without knowing what these primary conditions for each of us are in the first place, we are starting from a huge disadvantage when it comes to negotiating good sex with others.

'Conditions for good sex' and maintaining desire

Later on in this book you will learn about the processes that make us want to repeat behaviour that has been rewarding, and how relevant this is to desire. You will also learn about the latest developments in sex science that keep sexual satisfaction and desire alive over the course of your life. An important aspect of understanding your own sexuality is recognizing that 'sex' is not just one thing, and the types of sex, the way you have sex, the pleasure you get from it and how it makes you feel about yourself and your relationship are all crucial factors in sexual satisfaction and desire. 'Sex' can mean any number of experiences day to day, year to year, or relationship to relationship, and it's important to understand what types of 'sex' are good for you and in what contexts. You can see this reflection as looking inwards at your own sexuality before we can consider how your sexuality fits with anyone else's, as it's essential to have a clear understanding of how your own sexuality operates before you can expect it to dovetail optimally with a partner's.

Often I use this 'conditions for good sex' triangle as a starting point in therapy, to help people get a basic understanding of which elements of their sex life are going well and which need further attention. We spend some time on each of the three aspects, writing the conditions that the person feels are important for them for psychological arousal and physical touch, and rating them according to how close they are to where they would like them to be in their most recent sexual encounters. We then spend some time considering indicators that they are in the moment, such as a feeling of transcendence or being completely absorbed in sensation or a partner's body to the exclusion of all else, or the types of thoughts or distractions that they find themselves plagued by.

We then move on to understanding the ways in which elements of the triangle impact on each other, and you'll learn exactly how these processes happen later on in this book. For example, distraction reduces our ability to experience sexual sensation. Being more turned on makes it more likely that we are absorbed in the moment. High levels of psychological arousal are great, but not if the touch is unpleasant, as then it will decline. High levels of psychological arousal and our preferred physical touch will have no impact if all we can focus on is what our thighs look like or whether the other person is thinking of their ex.

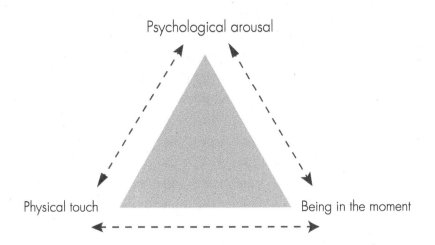

CONDITIONS FOR GOOD SEX

Psychological arousal

Physical touch

Being in the moment

I might use the 'conditions' triangle to help people reflect and make sense of their sex life currently. Sometimes we discover that their physical needs aren't being met, as their partner doesn't know what they like (or does know, but just doesn't do it). Sometimes they don't feel safe to let themselves go with the person they are with. Other times the environment they are mostly having sex in is deeply unerotic or distracting. Often, their mind is elsewhere, and without your brain involved, sex can feel like you're going through the motions. Mapping out this 'conditions' triangle once for partnered sex, and once for masturbation, can also be really eye-opening, as it becomes apparent how much having difficulty being in the moment, or getting the touch that works best for you, may be with partners only. This might be, for example, because sex with someone else is full of distracting thoughts about being judged. Or perhaps psychological arousal is at its highest with a partner as opposed to masturbation, as you struggle to generate fantasy or recall hot memories alone and feel you need the presence of someone else to be really turned on?

There are no rights and wrongs with the preferences that people have, and all (consensual) sexual preferences and expression are valid. Also, this 'conditions for good sex' triangle must be seen as a snapshot in time, rather than a template for life, as our sexual preferences, wants, needs and confidence are in constant flux. For this reason, if you would like to have a go at mapping this out for yourself, I would suggest you repeat the exercise periodically, as your needs and wants will change. You can use it to reflect on how much of the time your conditions for good sex are met both when you're alone (solo sex) and when you are with a partner. At the end of this chapter you'll find a guide to getting started mapping this out for yourself.

LUCY'S CONDITIONS FOR GOOD SEX WITH A PARTNER

Physical touch – likes kissing, starting off sensual and moving to deep, passionate kissing, soft gentle touch to the body but not squeezing or grabbing, likes indirect touch to the clitoris through her underwear or by pressing down on the pubic mound, dislikes direct touch, especially if the clitoris is exposed. Likes being on top of her partner due to the indirect clitoral stimulation it offers.

Psychological arousal – likes casual sex, where she gets to explore new bodies and be completely herself with someone who doesn't know her, likes novelty of a new partner and prefers sex where there is power play involved somehow. Finds looking at chests/shoulders a turn on, likes sex in luxurious surroundings, enjoys risk, likes to see desire on their faces, enjoys talk during sex about what's happening/what they want, likes sex that makes her feel 'free' to ask for what she wants, likes to feel in control.

Being present – mostly feels completely absorbed in the moment but is sometimes distracted by thoughts about the environment, how into it they are, how her stomach looks and whether this is what the other person wants.

Learning about sex, in terms of the sex positive, neutral or sex negative messages we have received, as well as our understandings about our own anatomy and sexual response are crucial foundations for a lifetime of sexual satisfaction. Also, for many of us, there is a gap in our knowledge about anatomy, pleasure and other factors which define and make sex feel good for us. This gap in knowledge is perpetuated by gender inequality and is demonstrated by the way women who have sex with men often enjoy less pleasure in the form of orgasms from sex than anyone else. Having a strong understanding of the psychological and physical aspects of what makes sex good for us and being able to be in the moment during sex are the starting points for having good sex with someone else. These conditions for good sex reflect the fact that sex is not just a physical experience that we do with our bodies, and that we all hold individual (and changing) preferences. Becoming more aware of this is an important precursor to being able to influence the sex we are having in a way that creates meaningful experiences and satisfaction. For many of us, there is a gap that has emerged between the sex neutral or sex positive starting point we need to enter into a sexual experience with, and the reality of our feelings about sex. Closing the gap by filling in these foundations is the first part of the journey.

Exercise:
Reflection – Understanding your own 'conditions for good sex' triangle

Draw a triangle on a large piece of paper and write the three headers 'psychological arousal', 'physical touch' and 'being present' on each point. Think back to the three best and three worst sexual experiences you have had with another person, and try to recall everything about these experiences that made them great (or not) for you in order to help you fill in each section.

After you have done this, add to the triangle anything you have not experienced in real life but feel you would like, as well as anything which works for you during masturbation, but less so with a partner. Try to make sure you have a good number of points under each. Below is a series of prompts which may help, though there is so much variety in 'conditions for good sex' that you should not be constrained by this list when coming up with your own.

- Feeling in sync with the other person

- Being able to ask for what you want

- Tension/build-up/erotic charge/suspense

- Making/hearing noise

- Sexual talk

- Visual cues like watching hips thrusting, seeing biceps rhythmically moving, seeing wetness, seeing body parts that are attractive

- Eye contact

- Environmental factors: lighting, music, surroundings, textures
- Body confidence
- Intimacy
- Having sex with more than one person
- Playing with power
- Playing with restraint or pain
- Biting
- Pushing boundaries
- Types of touch: gentle, firm, grabbing, slapping, stroking,
- Types of kissing and places you like to be kissed
- Taking control / relinquishing control
- Positions (not just sexual positions – positions you like to be in for kissing, for example)
- Sex acts (giving or receiving oral sex, fingers inside vagina / anus, rimming, penetrative vaginal / anal sex, rubbing bodies up close together, etc)
- How you like to feel about yourself / see yourself during sex
- How you like to experience the other person and how they act during sex
- Attraction to the person
- Animalistic / passionate sex
- Feeling free / alive / spiritual

Trying it out – sharing this with a partner

If you've been able to complete this for yourself and are in a relation-ship, a great next step is to be able to share it with a partner. In an ideal world, you would get them to read this section of the book and complete theirs too. Then, when you have the time and energy to sit down together and discuss them, do so, using the principles of:

➲ Listening well and asking probing questions, i.e. 'What do you mean by this one?'

➲ Not ridiculing or judging each other's conditions

➲ Making an attempt not to get defensive or into an argument

➲ Being careful with the words you use to discuss them: go gently

Once you have compared these (and remember that they are a snapshot in time, not a definite map for your lifelong sexuality), discuss the following:

1) Is there anything on your partner's 'conditions' triangle that you didn't know before? Ask them more about it. Is this something you might agree to try out/build on?

2) For the things that you did know, how often do these things feature in your sex life? If they're infrequent, what gets in the way?

3) There will be differences between your 'conditions' triangle and theirs. This is normal and not a sign of sexual incompatibility. There will be some total 'no-no's, which neither of you feels you want to incorporate, and this is fine. But are there any that, with some modification, you'd be prepared to look at further? For example, you might not be into kissing with tongues but your partner might be. Try asking them what it is that they like about

this. Perhaps it's that this type of physical contact represents *passion* to them? If so, is there another type of kiss, such as rough or deep kissing, that would work instead? Or you might decide that, although tongues is not your thing, you'd be happy to do it from time to time, especially if it's a big deal for them? I'll introduce you to the concept of 'sexual giving', in terms of the impact of being generous in this way has for long-term sexual satisfaction later on in this book.

Two
The Truth About Sex and Desire

4

Sex in our society

I mentioned in the last chapter that often, when we think about sex, we think of it as a biological or, perhaps, relational phenomenon – that sex happens *in our bodies* and/or *between us and other people*. In my experience of talking with thousands of people about their sex lives and what is working or not working for them, I notice that it is much harder for us to recognize the impact of family, culture, society and language on our sex lives. The impact of these factors is almost so large that the boundaries are outside of our field of vision and so it's difficult for us to spot the weight they carry.

Let's take Cara, for example. Cara came to see me and described some unsatisfactory sexual experiences, as well as a history of painful sex, difficulty with orgasms and an experience of being able to take or leave sex, which was showing itself in very little sense of desire. She was a twenty-something white heterosexual woman, originally from the UK, and she'd started having sex at university, initially delaying having penetrative sex because she felt it was the right thing, for her, to preserve her virginity. This was all connected to growing up in a family where sex was not talked about, and pleasure-giving body parts, such as the clitoris, were not named. When sex *was* referenced, the subtext was that it was something that 'good girls don't do' or should be frightened to do, as 'so much can go wrong'.

To delay losing her virginity, Cara felt she needed to avoid all sexual encounters with men, as she told me that 'it's unfair to lead men on', 'they get carried away' and 'it's not right to expect to do some things but not penetrative sex'. Because of this, and also her negative view of masturbation, she went into her first sexual experience, aged twenty, armed with very little knowledge of her own anatomy and sexual needs, and a sense of 'giving away' her virginity in a sexual act that she felt was overdue and was all about what men needed. Cara described finding her experiences of sex to date unarousing, uncomfortable and, on occasion, wanting her partners to stop but having a strong sense of 'we've started so I'll let them finish'. Her sexual encounters so far had been mostly negative or neutral, and were based on the following internalized beliefs:

- ✪ wanting or enjoying sexual pleasure is shameful, especially for women

- ✪ sex is about men's needs more than women's

- ✪ women are the gatekeepers but not the drivers of sexual activity

- ✪ women's sexual pleasure is less important than men's, especially when it comes to casual sex

- ✪ for women, looking good and a partner's satisfaction are more important than personal satisfaction

- ✪ it's not desirable for women to direct the sexual experience in relation to their wants and needs

- ✪ once you've started down a particular route, it would be impolite to stop

For Cara, none of these beliefs (which are entirely rooted in social norms and scripts around sex, gender politics and British values) were immediately obvious to her as contributors to her current difficulties. Instead, she had come to see me as she felt she was a woman who had difficulties with having orgasms, painful sex and low desire. But these sexual problems are not located *within* Cara. Cara would have not had these same sexual difficulties in another context (for example, if she had been male, or if she identified as a lesbian) because these difficulties are mostly rooted in heterosexual scripts and the playing out of these scripts in real life. This doesn't mean that Cara wouldn't have had any difficulties with sex, just that it's unlikely that they would have been the same ones. Re-read the bullet points above, imagining that Cara was male, and see where you think she'd be at with her experience of pleasure or desire.

But where have these internalized beliefs about sex come from? And why would Cara then attribute these sexual problems to there being something wrong with her, rather than reject these unhelpful societal ideas and refuse to settle for this kind of sex?

The role of social norms in shaping our sex lives

Social psychologists explain how we behave in relation to others and why. They use cornerstone psychological theories, such as conformity, compliance, social learning and identification theory, to explain, on a social level, why we do what we do. These theories basically translate to a human desire to fit in, belong, learn from what we see, make classifications of ourselves and others, outline the characteristic of certain groups (such as 'female', 'Western', 'Muslim', 'young') and the efforts we then make to adopt the characteristics of groups we identify with, to 'toe the line'. None of us exist in a vacuum and, whether we like it or not, we experience a gravitational pull to do what's expected of us, adhere to social norms and behave in a certain way.

Social psychology theories explain the dynamics between groups and how these dynamics can result in discrimination, stereotypes and injustice, and how we can risk exclusion or disapproval from other group members if we don't respect these social rules and scripts. They also explain how the world around us teaches us how we should be through how others behave and what we see in the media. Essentially, we learn by what we see and what we understand is deemed acceptable for our identity.

Consider masculinity as an example. Being 'one of the lads' or being told to 'man up' in response to displaying emotion or sensitivity is one way some members of the social group of 'male' might respond to another member acting in a way they feel threatens the status or integrity of that group, as the group has historically had a core perceived characteristic of 'being tough'. The social group 'male' also has a historically elevated and privileged social status based on a belief that 'masculinity (which = toughness) is superior' that it doesn't want to risk losing.

Concepts of social psychology are crucial when it comes to understanding sex and why we do the things we do. This is because, firstly, even though the ideas we get from the world around us about sex are not 'truths', they are so strongly socially enforced that they feel like they are, so we don't often question them or notice their impact. Secondly, given we learn how to 'be' sexual from our family of origin and from the world around us, we develop a perception of how sex should look and boundaries for behaviour deemed acceptable for our age, gender expression, race, sexuality, religion and cultural group. All of this learning filters down into the nuts and bolts of how we are sexual with others, helping or hindering us, mostly without us even realizing. This is what we'll unpick in this chapter. My aim is to raise your awareness of the impact of societal messages or norms on your sex life, with the aim of encouraging you to take action in rejecting the pull of any influences you are not happy with.

How we learn about sex

Within families, learning about sex starts as soon as we are born. In Chapter 3, we touched upon how we learn from the way our care-givers talk (or crucially, don't talk) about pleasure, genital anatomy and sex. For example, we learn about how much power we have over our right to bodily autonomy by not being always able to say no, even when we don't want to do to something we're being asked to do with our bodies, such as kissing a relative, or finishing all the food on our plate. This kind of learning teaches us that the social rules of politeness and convention outweigh our personal physical or psycho-logical discomfort in favour of someone else's needs.

Through consistent positive or negative comments about our appearance we learn from family members how important it is for girls to 'look nice', and how this is often prioritized over values, inter-ests or worldviews. From the use of often gender-specific language, such as 'bossy', for example, we learn that it's not seen as desirable for people identifying as female to be assertive, which is a real disad-vantage when it comes to sex. Social learning theory (learning through seeing and imitating) shows us how what we are exposed to about how adults 'do' relationships and sexuality, and what we absorb from this, makes a significant difference to how we ourselves 'do' sex and relationships as we grow.

We also know that, by primary school age, children have strongly held ideas about gender, with girls falsely perceiving themselves as physically weaker, less destined for success and having more responsibility to 'look pretty' than boys.[1] This might, at first, sound like it's relatively unconnected to our sex lives, but it is most definitely not, as this concept of women as 'less than' paves the way for the patriarchal society we live in that disadvantages women's sex lives in later years.

It doesn't take a great leap to see how early learning such as this can play out unhelpfully in sexual situations later on. In these early years, we may learn that sex equals shame, that sex is wrong or that our role in sex is to please others, look good and manage our inner discomfort silently. The impact of this kind of learning, especially on women, is why a commitment to lifelong sex positive education is so crucial.

Understanding the powerful role of social leaning and norms with regards to sex and how this intersects with gender (plus other contexts, such as race) is crucial to understanding our relationship with desire. Let me explain how.

Sexual Script Theory[2] describes the way in which societal and cultural expectations around sex shape our behaviour and interactions by providing us with clear expectations and boundaries to adhere to. These expectations are heavily gendered and shaped by the media, language, and interactions we have with others. Sexual Script Theory is the playing out of social psychology in our sex lives. Although the word 'script' implies that these ideas are explicit – and they can be at times, in the language we use – they are just as often implicit, alluded to by stories in the media, folklore and social convention.

The pervasiveness and impact of sexual scripts have been heavily researched, both in terms of how much they are replicated in the media and cultural messages and how people of all genders subscribe to them. Here are a few of the dominant sexual scripts in Western societies that have been identified as widespread and impacting on people's behaviour:[3]

- Men are sexual subjects with desires to be acted on and women are sexual objects who gain gratification from being desired

- Men have higher levels of sexual desire and 'uncontrollable' sexual impulses

- It's more important that men orgasm in heterosexual sex

- Penetrative vaginal sex is the most important sexual act in heterosexual sex

- Motherhood and getting older mean a woman should be less sexual

- Men show masculinity through high desire and many partners and women show femininity by sexual restraint

- Women should be less sexually assertive and initiate sex less

- Women feel that they should perform during sex in a way that increases men's sexual attraction to them and prioritizes men's sexual pleasure

- Heterosexual sex ends when men come

- Women are more motivated by relationship intimacy and closeness in sex than pleasure

- Women have an obligation to comply with their partner's need for sex to maintain relationship satisfaction

- Women's orgasms are more challenging to achieve than men's

And there are many more, including some particularly interesting ones relating to reciprocity in regards to oral sex, and also some specific ones for women who have sex with women, which we'll come to.

Sexual Script Theory proposes that, if we choose to go against these implicit social 'rules', there are sanctions which manifest as disapproval from others and which risk the individual who transgresses being labelled as problematic and less desirable. This is borne out in research when people are given scenarios related to the scripts above and then asked to judge people who deviate from them. People displaying behaviour outside of these scripts are judged more harshly and labelled less desirable – for example, women who are sexually assertive. There is evidence to suggest that these scripts might hold more weight in casual sexual encounters or at the start of relationships than they do in longer-term relationships, but the influence of them for all of us remains on some level, whether we feel constrained by them at this present moment or not.

You might feel as though you are aware of these scripts but do not believe in them or go along with them in your sex life. Great! Being aware of such influences is crucial to being aware of the contribution they have and making attempts to resist what's unhelpful, but it's often not as simple as this. As I mentioned, social norms make it very difficult for us to break free of the 'rules' that we are led to believe we should all adhere to, by creating sanctions which kick in as a result of perceived transgressions. We only need to look at the #MeToo movement to see the widespread prevalence of women being treated as objects for another person's gratification. We hear the atrocious stories of women accused of 'leading men on' when they dressed in a certain way and then changed their minds about a sexual encounter or stopped showing enthusiastic consent. There is still too much injustice related to the people who perpetrate these crimes not being held to account because of constructs such as 'boys will be boys' or it being 'just locker-room talk'. The ramifications of these sexual scripts are dominant, widespread, dangerous and, sadly, affect many of us whether we like them/believe in them or not.

The impact of the privilege and personal agency that women have is crucially relevant here. Not all women have equal agency, privilege and resources and we mustn't presume that they do. Race, religion, culture and economics play a part in how women are seen sexually as well as how able and safe women feel to overtly reject the impact of these scripts or not. Sexual scripts might be highly gendered, but the impact of them between women is partially connected to the intersection of other contexts.

Sexual scripts for women who have sex with women, in some ways, provide more sexual freedom. There is not, for example, a typical script for what lesbian sex should look like in terms of who does what and in what order. This is in contrast to women who have sex with men, who will often give a set description of how sex should typically look in formulaic order. Although this is partially why women who have sex with women typically have higher levels of sexual satisfaction, if you're about to have sex with another woman for the first time, the absence of a script can be confusing and scary. While largely unhelpful, one of the theories behind why we have societal scripts is that they reduce anxiety by providing us with information about how we should behave in social situations.

Also, living in a heteronormative world (heteronormative meaning everyone is presumed straight, and language, institutions and culture are geared towards this) means that, however you identify your sexual orientation, it doesn't stop you being continually exposed to heterosexual sexual scripts. The impact of this for women who have sex with women shows itself in a different way. Firstly, by leading to a sense of your sex life not 'fitting in', being afraid to hold hands in public or being asked inappropriate questions about how your sex life can possibly work. Secondly, how you make sense of how to 'be' in a sexual relationship with another woman when our sexual scripts position men as the initiators and performers of sex, with high levels of desire, and women as passive recipients.

The impact of these scripts was never more evident than during the 'lesbian bed death' era. 'Lesbian bed death' was a term used colloquially and in the scientific community in the 80s to refer to the fact that is was presumed (based on scripts that women were inherently less sexual, low in desire and passive sexually) that women who have sex with women would eventually stop having sex after a certain period of time together.

Of course, we now know that this isn't true. The desire of women in same-sex relationships works in the same way as with women who have sex with men, meaning that many women in long-term relationships might report low spontaneous desire, if you ask them how often they think and feel about sex out of the blue, and this in itself is not problematic. Recent studies comparing the sex lives of women in same-sex and mixed-sex relationships have once and for all put the 'lesbian bed death' myth, well, 'to bed'[4]. But, despite 'lesbian bed death' being discredited as a phenomenon, it still lingers as a sexual script for women in same-sex relationships and, sadly, can sometimes stop women who have sex with women making changes to their sexual relationship if they start to feel unhappy with how sex is going, as they (incorrectly) fear it is just the start of an inevitable decline.

One of the things we do know is that for women in same-sex relation-ships their desire is negatively affected by how impacted they are by heterosexism in society and the 'minority stress' it causes.[5] 'Minority stress' refers to being part of a marginalized group and the fear of coming out or being visible in relation to this, along with the psychological toll it takes at times to hide who you are. This means that, for women who identify as lesbian or bi, connecting with the wider LGBT community, coming out to trusted others and finding places to socialize and feel safe are key not just to mental health but to sexual satisfaction and desire too.

Our heteronormative society is also responsible for the script that 'being straight is normal and best', and this is conveyed in everyday language, social conventions and institutions. Despite increasing 'minority stress' for non-hetero people, this script is also damaging to a much larger body of people than those who currently identify as LGBT. The reason being that science tells us that sexual orientation in humans is unlikely to be binary (that is, straight or gay) and that most people will fall somewhere in the middle (remember Kinsey?). It's the sexual script that 'straight = best', plus the influence of homophobia (often stemming from a fear of transgressing this purported norm), that stops more people from exploring this side of their sexual self, exploration that could lead to higher levels of sexual authenticity, satisfaction and desire. How might living in a society that isn't largely homo/bi-phobic change how you consider your sexual experiences or expression? A percentage of you reading this might feel more comfortable (even in a small way) to explore a side of yourself that you currently don't feel able to, as it transgresses social convention and risks your membership of the social group of heterosexual. It's important to remember what we explored in Chapter 1: that the marginalization of same-sex activities has not always been problematic in the UK, and certainly isn't in all cultures and communities across the world, but is an unfortunate example of our historical classification of 'homosexuality' as a mental disorder and illegal, amongst other things.

Penis-in-vagina sex is 'real sex' – the ultimate unhelpful heterosexual script

If I were to ask Cara why she opted to have penetrative sex as part of her sex life, given that she didn't feel she got anything from it and she found it uncomfortable, I guarantee she would look at me as if I had just arrived from Mars. Heterosexual sex has such a set script of penis-in-vagina sex being 'real sex' that couples feel they can't imagine a sexual relationship without it, or imagine their partners would leave them if they insisted on dropping it. I'm not for one second suggesting we should abandon PIV sex altogether, just wanting to demonstrate that some of our sexual scripts are so pervasive and dominant that even the thought of deviating from them seems absurd, and it's this feeling that pulls us back in line with the 'shoulds' of social convention.

The influence of the media on how we see sex

In the UK, we typically spend around nine hours a day interacting with digital media, roughly half of which is TV, and the other half online digital content and social media.[6] It's a known and well-proven fact that what we see, and read about, in the media influences our beliefs, attitudes and behaviours (including sexual scripts). There are a multitude of media messages out there for us to pick up on, such as how our bodies should look or that periods are something that shouldn't be talked about openly, the judgement that comes down on people who are unfaithful in monogamous relation-ships or that penis size is important, how much sex we should be having, etc., etc.

All of these messages impact on our attitudes and behaviour, causing us to fear the judgement of our social group and identity if we transgress them. This happens with all dominant messages that we are exposed to through the media – for example, messages around food. But there is something unique about sex. With food and diet, it's likely that you are constantly exposed to adverts showing tasty food, say, pizza or ice cream, on TV, as well as conflicting messages about body image dictating what your body must look like to be 'good enough'. With food, you will be able to balance any conflicting messages you are exposed to with first-hand knowledge of seeing how and what your family eat, talking with them openly about what they eat and why, or even hearing them talk about their relationship to food.

Sex is so different because there's often such an absence of sex-related conversation in our lives. The consequence of this can be that, when it's not talked about openly and honestly, when we see it on TV it's often the first time we've seen it, and the most times we'll ever see people other than ourselves do it. So, in the absence of open conversation elsewhere, we grab hold of that information and absorb those messages in what we see about how sex is as absolute fact. The absence of talking about the truth of sex in our families, schools and society in general makes the media representations of how sex happens and how sex should be even more powerful.

Think about the last sex scene you saw on TV or in a film. It was probably between a (cis) man and woman, it probably involved sexual acts based on this predefined sexual script (mainly kissing and penetrative vaginal sex) and it would have included very little of anything else.

The scene would also likely have included a sex scene that was high in spontaneous passion, where both partners felt a sudden urge to connect sexually at the same moment and in the same way. This representation of desire is what we are used to seeing on TV and in films: spontaneous, mutual, synchronized passion. It's no wonder we feel despondent when our own sex lives don't match up. Where is the TV/film representation of a couple who negotiate sex, as one of them feels like it and the other doesn't? Who start off not feeling that into it and passion builds as their arousal does? Who look at each other and say, 'Will we regret it if we don't do the housework and just have sex instead?' I have seen these representations on TV at times, but they often act as an indicator of sexual problems to the viewer rather than being represented for what they are: a normal, well-functioning long-term sexual relationship.

Of course, there are many couples who have been together a very long time who still look at each other with desperate lust, and have moments of perfectly synchronized spontaneous passion – and I wouldn't want to perpetuate the myth that this is not possible in long-term relationships as it *most definitely is*. But this same couple may also have moments where sex is less erotic, more negotiated, less sparky, and the point here is that they could be forgiven for worrying that there is something wrong with this type of sex, given the lack of exposure we have to it. We don't have a script for this.

As I mentioned, the type of sex we usually see on TV often consists of a bit of kissing, quickly followed by vaginal penetration and quick mutual orgasm in positions where any kind of clitoral stimulation is unlikely. This repetitive exposure to 'how sex looks' is one of our forms of sex ed and one of the important ways our sexual scripts are perpetuated. One consequence of this is that we start to see what is represented on screen as the norm, and view our inability to reach orgasm in this quick and easy way as a failing in comparison (hence faking it, as an obvious and common solution). I mentioned earlier that I have women come to see me with problems with orgasm who, it turns out, can orgasm just fine from oral sex or masturbation but not from penetrative sex. This near-constant representation of an impossible goal of women orgasming from two minutes of penetrative sex with virtually no build-up has created a sense that women's bodies are faulty when they don't oblige in the same way, especially when you consider that most women can't orgasm like this to begin with.

Porn and sexual scripts

When it comes to porn, I feel strongly about two things. Firstly, the idea that porn is harmful, wrong or always degrading to women is untrue. Porn as an industry is as large as the television industry and, just as you see the full range, from poor quality, unethical or degrading TV shows to high quality, ethically produced and empowering TV on mainstream television, you see the same range in porn. The problem is that when we think or talk about porn, we are often talking about mainstream/free porn, which is just one section of the porn market. It is certainly true that there are some parts of the industry which use terminology, practices or storylines which are degrading to women, perpetuate unhelpful ideas about how sex should look and are of dubious ethics. But there are also many porn producers making ethical content which privileges things like diversity, autonomy, equal pleasure and consent.

Despite the variety in porn, it's certainly the case that mainstream free porn is easily accessible, heavily viewed by people of all genders, and that the adult entertainment industry is one of the fastest growing sectors.[7] We also know that a large proportion of young people in the UK have seen porn by their early teens and that this is most likely to be mainstream porn. As we have already discussed, in the absence of good sex education, TV in general and porn in particular can be ways young people learn about sex. But how has increasing access to porn shaped our sexual scripts? And is this something to worry about?

One of the changes in sexual behaviour picked up by Natsal 3 was a rising trend for younger generations of heterosexuals to include anal sex as part of their sexual practice, in comparison to older generations (17% of 16–24-year-old women have had anal sex in the last year, compared with 8% of 45–55-year-olds).[8] One possible explanation for this increased trend is that younger Brits are more open and liberal about sex, meaning that they are more likely to try a sexual practice that has historically been more taboo during heterosexual sex. It's also possible that our sexual scripts are shifting as a result of the impact of mainstream porn, where there is a growing trend for showing anal penetration as a standard part of heterosexual sex. Our choice to have anal sex might therefore be our version of doing what we think society and our partners expect of us as part of 'normal' sex. There's nothing wrong with anal sex, of course, but what is important is that how we see sex shifts depending on what we are exposed to, whether that's the more relaxed attitude of our peers, or exposure to new sexual scripts in porn.

One of the other concerning trends with mainstream porn is its lack of attentiveness to female sexual pleasure. Research published in *The Journal of Sex Research* by Seguin and colleagues in 2017 reviewed the fifty most viewed Pornhub videos of all time and analysed them for orgasm-inducing sexual acts (such as clitoral stimulation) as well as how often they contained visual and verbal representations of women's sexual pleasure. Of them, only 18% showed visual or verbal cues suggesting women's orgasm, compared to 78% showing men's.[9] In these videos, the presence of dominant sexual scripts was noted in the (incorrect) portrayal of most women orgasming from penetration, the presentation of sexual acts based on female sexual pleasure as 'added extras', and the focus on male orgasm as both more important and signifying the end of sex.

Porn is not the source of our sexual dissatisfaction, but unless we become more porn literate (and teach our children to be so also), or until ethical porn becomes more mainstream, porn will continue to take an ill-placed spot centre stage in our sex education and potentially contribute to the evolution of our sexual scripts over time.

So why is this important?

The recognition that social and cultural factors shape our sex lives as much as (and perhaps more than) what happens in our bodies and relationships opens up huge possibilities for our enjoyment of sex and our experience of desire. Widening our field of vision and spotting the influence of society in this way also changes the location of a problem with desire. Remember that 34% of women in the UK have experienced a lack of interest in sex in the last year, that pleasure from sex is often missing for women (as evidenced by the orgasm gap) and that women have been raised not to be assertive sexually, not to put their own needs first and to make sure they look nice above all else. How can we overlook the influence of this on desire? Desire is difficult to cultivate and maintain in these contexts.

How can we not locate at least part of any problems we might have with sex here?

I should say, by the way, that men are also hugely disadvantaged by the pervasiveness of these dominant sexual scripts, as they create perceptions of masculinity which suggest that men are sex-crazed, intimacy-averse, bold sexual initiators, low in self-control, which (as well as not being factually correct) causes its own problems for men's sex lives. But that's not the focus of this book and, when it comes to sex, women, particularly straight women, get the roughest end of the deal from society by far.

Let's revisit Cara for a second. What might Cara's experience of sex have been like if she had known more about her own pleasure? If she had understood that she was entitled to enjoy any type of sex she wanted on her own terms? If she felt she never had to have penetrative sex again and that this was perfectly fair on her sexual partners? If she felt her desire and need for sexual release were just as powerful, or more powerful, than a man's? If she dominated the sexual experience and therefore made it entirely focused on her wants? I can tell you the answer to this, if you're not there already. Cara would not have been sitting opposite me, seeking my help.

Imagine Cara was raised in a family culture where she was encouraged to seek pleasure, enjoy her body and have no shame in either of these things. She might have enjoyed masturbation as part of her early sexual experiences and, as a result, learned exactly how she liked to be touched. Her lack of shame in talking about sex and the messages in her culture that women should ask for what they want sexually, might have led her to seek out sexual experiences where she could explore what she liked with someone else. In these experiences she would have been clear, direct and assertive, saying things like

'I'd like you to go down on me then penetrate me with your fingers just before I come', and she wouldn't feel self-conscious about the lack of penetrative sex for them, the 'sidelining' of their pleasure for hers, or what they would think about her asking so directly. If she did have penetrative sex, it's likely that she would feel no pain, as she would be turned on (a direct result of being able to be sexually assertive and communicate one's needs) and she would feel confident and in control of the pace and speed of penetration. However, you can be sure that she would feel able to say 'I'd like to stop now please' at the point at which she got bored of, or felt discomfort with, penetrative sex, and she would not worry about the impact of this on her partner, or that it would jeopardize the future of the relationship. She might not feel constrained to stop at one orgasm either, even after her partner had come.

So ... Here's the challenge. We know from research that sexual assertiveness and autonomy are associated with higher levels of sexual satisfaction in relationships and sexual wellbeing.[10] In contrast, we also know that sexual submission and over-focus on a partner's pleasure to the exclusion of your own results in lower levels of sexual satisfaction and sexual functioning. But I have rarely met a heterosexual couple whose sex life has not been negatively affected by the scripts we have discussed in this chapter. I've also rarely met a heterosexual couple who have come to a first session with me having really reflected on the nuts and bolts of how sex happens and, crucially, which partner's needs are currently being served best as the backdrop to their sexual problems. Usually, there has been a lot of talk about sex, but mainly focused on the female partner's 'low' desire and how it can be fixed. The impact of society and culture on one partner's sexual needs being disadvantaged over another's is almost too large for them to be able to spot.

Dan and Vanessa had been together eleven years and came to see me as they both felt Vanessa's desire had dwindled to the point that it had become non-existent. When we talked about their sexual preferences and sexual history, I discovered that (like most women) Vanessa mostly enjoyed clitoral stimulation as her main source of sexual pleasure. In fact, when she masturbated, she did this using her hand, or a suction-type vibrator to stimulate her clitoris, and penetrating herself as part of masturbation simply never crossed her mind. Although it wasn't something she did often, she experienced high arousal and high pleasure from masturbating. When Dan and Vanessa had sex together, they had got into a habit of this being a couple of minutes of kissing, then Vanessa giving Dan oral sex, then him penetrating her, which lasted until he orgasmed. This sexual encounter is largely based on societal scripts we've discussed here – of what heterosexual sex *should* look like – and is mainly focused on Dan's sexual pleasure and experience. It's not that Dan is intentionally orchestrating sex which limits Vanessa's pleasure, or that Vanessa has even thought about the fact that this habit of sex is way off the mark when it comes to her pleasure. After all, they are both just recreating an image of sex that is societally constructed and *looks like sex to them*. They have seen it happening on TV this way a million times. It's what sex looks like to them. But when we look at what Vanessa is expected to get from this encounter in terms of physical reward, it is unsurprising that her arousal, enjoyment and desire have dwindled over time, and they're unlikely to flourish without this being addressed.

Inequality and the curse of the heterosexual sexual script

In my experience, it's really common for heterosexual couples like Vanessa and Dan to fall into a 'set menu' when it comes to sex.

This generally looks like a starter that's of a bit of a quick fumble, then a main course of penetrative sex. I often say it's better to think of sex as a buffet. You can have whatever you want in any order. It doesn't need to include the same things every time, or end with the same dish. Imagine how much more novel and exciting that would be.

LGBT couples often do this as standard and report much less predictable sexual encounters than their straight counterparts. If you were to adopt this idea in your own sex life, for example, sex could be kissing for a long time then ending in both of you giving and receiving oral sex. Sex could be both of you being sexual together with no penetration and no orgasms, or entirely focused on one of you with no touch at all to the other.

Sex can be whatever you want.

The Natsal data we reviewed in Chapter 2 tells us that there is a correlation between having genital contact without penetrative sex and better sexual function. It's possible that having very 'samey' sex every time you have sex lowers your sexual functioning by being so predictable, and/or couples with lower levels of sexual functioning have less of other types of sex, as things haven't been going so well. Either way, it's important to pay attention to the dangers of always 'ordering the set menu' if we want sexual satisfaction long term. Especially if you're planning on eating in the same restaurant every night for the rest of your life.

We live in a society where we are constantly striving for equal rights for women in all kinds of areas, but we are massively lagging behind when it comes to sex. Heterosexual women are often having the types of sex that are not the ultimate fit for their anatomy, then feeling shame and guilt for not experiencing the 'right amount' of pleasure or orgasms from those experiences, or experiencing a knock-on effect on their desire for sex with their partner, without even realizing these limiting and dissatisfying scripts are to blame.

This is why Cara is sitting in my room.

Faking orgasms and sexual scripts

We know that women fake orgasms frequently (roughly 50–65% of women report having faked or regularly fake orgasms) and for a variety of reasons[11] such as:

- wanting to look like a 'good sexual partner'

- wanting sex to end

- to protect a partner's feelings

- an attempt to enhance sex for them or their partner

- to avoid conflict or explanation

- wanting to prevent a partner from leaving

- to avoid shame, as they feel they should have come

Faking orgasms reinforces the sexual scripts we currently have available to us by creating the illusion that women are just as satisfied by the way sex is happening as men are. Faking it also affirms the false belief held by society that most women can come from penetrative sex. Faking it also does men a disservice, as it provides unhelpful feedback about the things that add to sexual pleasure and leads to unrealistic expectations – in fact, studies have found that men consistently overestimate the amount of women who reach orgasm and underestimate the amount of women who don't.[12] Faking orgasms is a key ingredient in the orgasm gap. But the frequency with which women are faking orgasms also tells us several important things about our current sexual scripts: women feel pressure to prioritize their partner's needs in such a way that it prevents communication about what *they* really want; women's pleasure is seen as an added bonus, not an expected essential; women find it hard to communicate that they want sex to stop in case they disappoint someone else. Faking orgasms is essentially a symptom of our current sexual scripts in action.

Reciprocity and oral sex in heterosexual scripts

In Chapter 2 we learned that certain sexual acts, like receiving oral sex, are often associated with pleasure and orgasms for women. So how does this fact show itself in social scripts around how (heterosexual) sex should look?

Fascinatingly, but frustratingly, we know that attitudes towards giving and receiving oral sex tend to see giving men oral sex as part of a duty that women should partake in, whether they enjoy doing it or not, whereas giving oral sex to women is seen as something that requires too much 'work' for men, is too much to ask for or asks for close up contact with our genitals in a way that we feel they (and perhaps we) won't feel comfortable with.

Research in the UK found that more than twice as many young people aged 16–18 expected men to receive oral sex as part of a sexual encounter as opposed to women (42% vs 20%),[13] and this disparity plays out in other countries, across sexual experiences and across the lifespan of partners. There is no doubt that pervasive societal negativity about the smell, appearance and taste of vulvas, combined with male sexual pleasure being seen as more important than women's, contributes to the sidelining of oral sex focused on women in heterosexual sex, and this has been described in research.

The widely held belief that giving oral sex is unpleasant for men combined with women's anxieties about the appearance, smell and taste of their vulva influences women to such an extent that *we* almost convince *ourselves* that we don't like it, *don't mind not having it* or *don't need it as part of our sex lives*. This, of course, is in contrast with the data that tells us it's one of the most pleasurable sexual acts for women. Feminist sex scientists and writers have long argued that holding on to these beliefs that it's *just not our cup of tea*, rather than a sexual double standard around inequity in relation to giving and receiving pleasure, acts as a smokescreen for a hard-to-swallow reality. Holding on to an idea that 'we just don't like it that much' allows us to maintain a sense that our sex lives are defined by equality and reciprocity in how sex happens when, in fact, they are not.

Perhaps you're wondering if another explanation for this inequity in receiving oral sex is that women just enjoy giving oral sex to men more than they do receiving it themselves? Afraid not. Many women report not liking or enjoying the sensation of giving oral sex or the taste of semen, but when asked why they do it, describe a strong social script that 'it's just what you have to do'. Incidentally, men report enjoying giving oral sex more than women report enjoying giving oral sex, which is another confusing piece of the puzzle when you consider that women do it at a rate of twice that of men AND that it's a more reliable route to orgasm for women than for men.

Sadly, it's more likely that the elevated importance of men's preferences and pleasure in our sexual scripts, our communal discomfort with women's genitals, and women's socialization to please, leads women to overlook these factors and perform oral sex much more frequently than men. If you are someone who avoids receiving oral sex but are not completely sure that you don't like it, rather you find it hard to feel entitled or be able to relax and enjoy it, perhaps it would be beneficial to experiment with this a bit? As with anything in life, the more we do something, the more comfortable we generally feel doing it, so whether it's about you changing your relationship with your vulva, getting reassurance from a partner about whether they enjoy giving oral sex and why, or just seeing if you can get more comfortable by doing it more, this could be a good thing for your sex life.

Women's bodies and society

Body image has a particularly important role to play in women's sexual confidence and experience of desire, and there have been many important studies that have demonstrated a strong relationship between the two. Whether it's our weight, shape, size, amount and location of body hair, how our vulva looks/smells/tastes or the size of our labia, we are plagued with worries about what sexual partners will think of our naked bodies.[14] Although body image concerns such as these are not unique to women, and more and more men are feeling insecure about their body image too, concerns about body image disproportionately affect women.

The process by which we are so impacted by concerns about how we look sexually is argued to be a byproduct of 'objectification theory'.[16] Objectification theory proposes that we have internalized the (very gendered) social scripts that self-worth is highly dependent on how we look. Therefore, when we feel we have to be naked in front of another person, we are overly focused on seeing our body from that other person's perspective and, in comparison to unrealistic societal expectations, we fear the judgement they may make of us. Being overly focused on body image in this way leads to us being distracted from sex, and we'll talk more about why this is crucial to enjoyment and desire in Chapter 6. For now, it's useful (though depressing) to know that poor body image is associated with lower sexual satisfaction, avoiding sex, struggling to have orgasms and having less desire to masturbate or have sex with a partner.[17]

There is no doubt whatsoever that how we feel about our bodies is one of the key culprits in regard to how we experience desire. The good news, though, is that the effects of body image concerns reduce for some women with length of relationship and age, meaning that, as time goes by in life generally or in a relationship, we may be less affected by such concerns.[18,19] The other good news is that, if this is the case for you, being aware of this and taking a position on it, as I will invite you to do at the end of this chapter, is a way of reducing the impact that it might be having on your sex life.

Mind your language

Language is both a key feature of society and a way in which our reality is created. When it comes to sex, the language we use has the opportunity to perpetuate unhelpful ideas and sexual dissatisfaction or, alternatively, set us and our desires free. Let's have a look at some of the ways language has been serving our sex lives badly so far.

I can't remember the last time I used the word *virginity*. Instead, I ask people about their first (consensual) sexual experience alone or with someone else as one of many key moments in their sexual history. Framing the start of our sex lives as an emerging sexual debut is also more inclusive of LGBT people, who may not have, or value, vaginal penetration as part of their sex lives in the same way. It also gets away from that horrible idea that we are giving away – instead of gaining – something precious that marks us out as ruined (women more than men) by someone else. I find throwing the word virginity in the metaphorical bin also very useful as a therapeutic intervention in its own right in sessions with clients. This is because, just by my choice of language, I can shift the value of penis-in-vagina sex from its pedestal of 'ultimate essential sex act' to just one of the things you might value in your sexual relationship, or even something which might be deeply unfulfilling to you that you are doing for someone else or because you think you should. The reason the word virginity is rated so highly as a construct in our society is because we have fallen into the trap of favouring penis-in-vagina sex as our 'definitive sex act' over all other types of sex, regardless of what we know to the contrary. For many women, other types of sex (including masturbation) feel more pleasurable, or more intimate, and are therefore arguably a better definition of sexual debut, but these sexual experiences are invisible in the language we have available to us in our society.

The same assumption behind the term virginity is also the reason that so many women in same-sex relationships get asked 'who's the man' or 'how on earth do you have sex'? The assumption is, if a penis doesn't go in a vagina, it isn't 'real sex'. It's an example of how narrow our sexual scripts can be and how they threaten to exclude a group who are perceived not to have access to this ultimate act (they, of course, do, but are not so foolish as to revere it over all else).

There's other language we use that adds to and fuels some of our less helpful social scripts. The concept of 'blue balls' – schoolyard slang for the idea that men's desire is so powerful that once they've started on the journey of arousal there will be health consequences if the destination of orgasm isn't reached – might be teenage talk, but it's fuel to those sexual scripts and is evident in my clinical work, where women frequently tell me that they feel that arousing their male partner and their partner not having an orgasm at the end of it is equivalent to their partner being hanged, drawn and quartered. You'll see the negative influence of this belief in Chapter 7, when we examine the impact of pressure on how women's desire works. What's often of interest, and reflects our scripts around women's desire, is that women very rarely have this same perception of their own arousal. They see it as entirely acceptable and expected that they should have to manage feelings of arousal that are left to dwindle away as their pleasure is sidelined. Nowhere is this more evident than the orgasm gap in casual sex, where, if you remember, women orgasm around 18% of the time with male partners. Women report that this is what they expect and accept. They don't worry about having 'blue labia', or that their genitals will combust or explode as a result of being turned on and not having a physical release. Our sexual scripts tell us that male sexuality and desire is more powerful and needs to be satiated, when, in fact, it is not.

Finally, the one word in our language I despise the most, which restricts our sexual pleasure and expression by its mere existence, is 'foreplay'. 'Sex' is any physical or psychological act that uses your body or mind for sexual pleasure or expression. I never use the word foreplay, as, to me, it represents the creation of a hierarchy through language that elevates some types of sex as 'better' or 'more like proper sex'. There are at least three main problems with the word foreplay:

1. It marks out one type of sex (PIV) as superior to all others and the 'main event', even though this type of sex benefits people with penises more than people with vaginas (see 'Orgasm Gap')

2. It suggests sex that follows a set formula, and predictability and lack of novelty are generally less exciting for sex for most people

3. It is not LGBT inclusive, as it suggests that much of the type of sex that LGBT people have is not 'real sex'

Please let's ditch 'foreplay' from our vocabulary and stop using it from this point on. Sex is so much more than that one act, and we'd all be better off if we started seeing and talking about it as such.

How we are our own worst enemy – the perpetuation of unhelpful societal beliefs

One of the many ironies of society is that we continue to support and perpetuate ideas about sex that cause us great misery, and we do so without questioning this. There are so many unhelpful ideas about sex that float around unchallenged that I could probably have written a whole other book full of them. I've picked a selection here that are some of my favourites to dismantle in sex therapy, as they are crucial to how we experience sex and desire in relationships.

The ease of spontaneous sex

We are led to believe that sex should happen spontaneously and easily without any considerable effort from anyone involved, and this is also linked with how we see sex happening on TV. It strikes me as odd that we often hear lots about the effort and investment people put into other areas of their life, such as to maintain a healthy diet or to stay fit, or when they want to create change or keep something to a certain standard, yet we often maintain a belief that sex should work just fine with zero effort or investment.

Connected to this is the idea that scheduling physical intimacy is unsexy. It's probably also related to the idea that 'good sex' should be spontaneous. I find this idea about planning being the antithesis of a good time really interesting, as it raises the question: what other enjoyable aspects of our life does planning lead to a lack of excitement or enjoyment? When you think about where you want to go on holiday, spend time considering where you want to go, imagine what it will be like, picture yourself there having a great time, imagining the sun on your skin, or how relaxed you'll feel, does that make the holiday less exciting or enjoyable? Would it be better if you didn't know you were going on holiday and you were ushered on to the plane at the last minute, not really sure where you are going, having not packed, not knowing whether you even feel like going on holiday or are ready for one at that moment?

I feel what people are really referring to when they recoil at the concept of scheduling is the idea that 'sex' being expected is off-putting, and in some ways this can certainly be true, as pressure and expectation can be real desire killers (more about this in Chapter 7). But there is a difference between carving out time for physical connection and pre-emptively consenting to sex you aren't even sure you want or will feel like, and it's a crucial one. Knowing that there is a no-pressure, enjoyment-filled, intimacy-fuelled fest planned that evening, which may lead to wanting more but also might not, can be really sexy. Also, knowing that this time is planned not only allows both of you to anticipate and fantasize about it (which are both important triggers for arousal and desire) but also allows you to put things in place which help with the practicalities of making it happen. This might be making sure you switch your phone off or resisting checking your stressful work emails, making an effort to be home from work on time, or not answering that call from your aunt which might take an hour. It might also lead you to take steps to connect with your own sexuality and do what you need to do to feel confident in your body. This might be having a shower, wearing something that makes you feel confident, or creating the right environment using music or temperature. If you reflect back to your 'conditions for good sex' triangle, there will be some clues here about what would help set the tone for you.

The other advantage of scheduled versus spontaneous physical intimacy is that it sets a tone of expectation between the two of you which allows you to flirt and build up anticipation throughout the day, amplifying each other's excitement (for example, sending a text 'How's your day?' 'A bit stressful TBH! Only thing getting me through is looking forward to chilling with you later ☺'. When it comes to sex, and the fact that it requires (at least) two people to be on the same page at the same time in this hectic modern age, why wouldn't we give ourselves the advantage of having the heads up that we are invested in creating a space for physical intimacy in which desire can flourish? Isn't this one of the most obvious way of helping each other and our sex lives along?

The three-times-a-week myth

One of my absolute favourite societal myths about sex and desire is that we should be having sex three times a week. I love this one mainly as a) it's so pervasive (it's what couples usually tell me they want their sex life to be), b) it's really far from how often we know couples are actually having sex (as you learned in Chapter 2), and c) it bears no relation to sexual satisfaction, desire or pleasure (the idea of frequency as a marker tells us nothing about our actual experience of sex). Nevertheless, it persists! I'm totally stumped about where this one comes from (tell me if you know!), but I do know it's quite resistant to extinction and it's the cause of an enormous amount of stress for a lot of people who feel their neighbours are beating them at meeting this magical number of three times a week.

Expect the worst for your sex life

Another unhelpful societal belief that I feel hinders sex in long-term relationships a great deal is the idea that there will be an inevitable decline in sexual satisfaction or passion. This saddens me, as once we subscribe to it, it can serve as a self-fulfilling hypothesis. Yes, for some couples, sex might start to lose its charm after a few years, due to normal changes in desire, or connected to changes in habits of how people relate as they get to know each other more, or linked with a change of circumstances, such as living together or having a child. But, sadly, the belief that this is the start of an inevitable decline is often the thing that stops couples doing something to rectify the situation. With knowledge and investment, desire can be sustained over many decades[20] and sexual satisfaction doesn't need to decline, even as a consequence of normal changes in desire over the course of a relationship. The secret to a good sex life in the long term is being able to discuss and adapt to the inevitable ebb and flow of desire and sex in a relationship. In Part Three we'll learn all about what makes sex good in the long term and how we can adopt these ideas and watch our sex lives flourish, even when life conspires against us. The problem is, as soon as we believe we are on an inevitable downward trajectory, with no escape and no hope, we stop making any attempt to adapt. How we evaluate our sex lives and what we believe about desire is crucial to how our sex lives then play out over time.

Dr Karen Gurney

Monogamy reigns supreme

Monogamy is possibly one of the best examples of a societal construct that influences our behaviour to such an extent that we find it hard to see it's there, instead imagining that being monogamous is just what humans do, and not a product of the influence of the religious, economic and political forces at work in our society, as mentioned in Chapter 1. What is fascinating about our (Western cultural) belief in the construct of monogamy is that not only does seeing humans as essentially monogamous lead us to expect that fidelity and satisfaction should come easily to us without effort, but we also end up with a great deal of societal disapproval of those who are seen to contravene it, whether they are content in their sexual relationships or not. I often feel that our acceptance of monogamy as inevitable and lifelong can be damaging to our sex lives, as it removes our sense of freedom to leave a relationship and can lead us to take a partner's long-term sexual interest and enthusiasm for granted, rather than seeing it as something to nourish. I'm certainly not anti-monogamy (or anti any relationship structure), but I am suggesting that it's useful to reflect on how we made the choice to be monogamous (did we, or are we just doing what's expected?). I'm also interested in how the social construct of monogamy being 'normal', or even 'easy if you love each other', helps or hinders our sex lives in terms of the effort we make to nurture it. For example, an expectation that monogamy is easy, natural and to be expected, even in the absence of a good sex life together, can be a dangerous assumption in a relationship, in my clinical experience. How might it impact on our investment in our sex lives if we saw monogamy as something which is not necessarily easy and, for many people, something that is dependent on relationship and sexual satisfaction?

Our intersectional identities and sex

In this chapter so far, I've spoken a great deal about the context of gender and the enormous impact of gender identity on how we think and behave in relation to sex. Gender is a hugely important construct, as not only is it one of the core constructs which shape how we see ourselves, but the social construction of gender in our society dictates how we are supposed to look, act, dress, behave, desire and 'do' sex. Similarly, the impact of gender politics on the act of sex itself is crucial to how we understand our sexual satisfaction and desire, as women's pleasure and desire are negatively impacted by restrictions on bodily autonomy, self-knowledge, assertion, pleasure, reciprocity and expectations to please.

I've also spoken about the context of sexuality, mainly as there is a large disparity between women who have sex with men and women who have sex with women regarding their experience of pleasure and satisfaction, which illustrates the huge impact of the context of gender and gender politics. But I have also referenced how the experience of having sex with men or having sex with women brings with it new opportunities and challenges for women in certain aspects of sex, such as the experience of pleasure, the pervasiveness of sexual scripts, gendered expectations about desire and the impact of living with heteronormativity/homophobia/biphobia/transphobia can have on how you feel or how you are treated with regards to your sexual expression.

But we mustn't assume that the contexts which make up our unique sexual history, understanding and experience stop at gender and sexuality, and it's crucial that we reflect on the other aspects of our identities that shape our lives and experience of the world, in turn making a difference to our experience of sex. For many of us, some of these contexts might feel even more influential to our relationship with sex and desire than sexuality or gender.

Earlier in this chapter we talked about the influence of the media and how our consumption of media impacts women's adherence to 'sexual scripts'. Much of this research (as with much of science) has been biased and focused on predominantly white women, and therefore doesn't take into account the different social and cultural factors or scripts that may be at play with the experience of race more widely. Recently, there have been some important attempts to redress this balance, and some newer studies have reported on key differences in the media impact on the sexual scripts available to women as they intersect with race.

We know that gendered sexual scripts are constraining and may be barriers to all women's sexual well-being, and it is argued that adhering to these sexual roles diminishes women's sexual entitlement and empowerment. However, we mustn't assume that women of colour are exposed to the same gendered scripts around sexuality as white women. There are key socio-historical differences informing how women of colour are judged, stereotyped and treated differently to white women around issues of sex and sexuality, due to the impact of racism in our society.

One example of this is a study which found that black women reported feeling concerned about asserting themselves and advocating for their own needs sexually for fear of reinforcing (harmful) negative stereotypes of black women as 'being overly sexual or animalistic'.[21] We can also see the influence of racism, oppression and violence with regard to women of colour in mainstream porn, where videos featuring a woman of colour are regularly titled with a reference to the fetishization of her race, or with a reference to the dynamics of her submitting to or being humiliated by a white man. It's these damaging ideas which lead to a society where sexual assaults on women of colour are tragically too common and are less likely to result in convictions.[22]

What's important here is that culture, society and our unique contexts have a far bigger influence on our individual experience of sex and desire than we might recognize. If we want to have a good relationship with sex and desire, we must pay attention to how who we are has shaped our social learning about the intersection of sex and race, culture, age, physical ability, body size/shape, class and religion.

The potential positive and negative impacts of all of these other contexts of our identities on sex are so large that they warrant a whole book (and there *are* many books devoted to each of them), so they are outside the scope of this chapter. Despite this, it can be really important to examine the role of the different contexts that make up who you are to work out which of the social messages about sex coming from these contexts you agree with or reject, which of them are in congruence and which clash, and which of them are helping or hindering your current sexual expression, including desire. At the end of this chapter there is an exercise to take you through this and make these implicit messages explicit, so that you can 'name the game' and feel more power over these messages than they currently have over you.

Given society has such a negative impact on our sex lives and desire, why don't we speak out about it more? Firstly, there are several things that we as a society simply do not talk about, and we therefore do not know about our own sexuality. We are not told much about how our bodies work, or that it's okay to ask for non-penetrative sex, or that other women feel the same way, that it's still 'sex' if you don't have penetration, that we're not unusual and that the odds are stacked against us to come in the way we're expected to, particularly if TV is anything to go by.

Secondly, we care too much. We care about being perceived as unusual, about moving too far from the norm, about a partner's pleasure or disappointment being more important than ours, and about rocking the boat. This is all understandable, as it's rooted in us as being social animals, with a desire to conform and fit in, as well as in persistent and detrimental gender politics at an institutional and linguistic level.

What's great about sex, though, is that, given I've just shared with you all the ways by which sex is a socially determined concept, it's also, therefore, something that can see shifts over time. These movements come with changes in dominant ideas, changes in how we use language, and as other cultural values (like alternative relationship structures, like feminism) shift with it. Despite the limits that our current societal beliefs place on our sex lives, we also know that these narratives and scripts have shifted in the last 100 years. Even in the last fifty. So, we can choose to rebel, choose not to conform, choose to speak up about what does or doesn't work for us. We can decide to reject the scripts and the constraining language that doesn't serve us. We can experiment with asking to do things differently and noticing the effects, on us, on our partners, on our mutual satisfaction and on our desire over time. We can add to the rewriting of these scripts.

Perhaps it's time we brought our politics to the bedroom?

Take home messages from this chapter

- Our society, culture and the interaction of this with our individual contexts (gender, race, sexuality, age) have a huge impact on our sex lives, often more powerfully than we are aware

- These sexual scripts and cultural norms can have both a direct and indirect impact on desire, by creating the illusion that desire is less powerful for women, by defining sex as something which doesn't always produce pleasure for us, or taking away our ability to be assertive

- Language is a key vehicle for sexual norms and maintains frameworks for sex that limit positive sexual experience and pleasure and create a narrow perception of 'sex'

- The media and porn have a large part to play in the maintenance of sexual scripts, and this becomes even more relevant in communities with poor sex education at home or in school

- Societal beliefs about sex for women are not uniform, and being black, gay, older or disabled will change the nature of the ideas about sex we are exposed to

- Despite not believing some of these ideas about sex or how we should behave in our society, we will be affected by them and might find ourselves going along with them more at certain stages of life (for example, accepting orgasm gaps in hook-up sex) or experiencing negative consequences for rebelling against them (for example, being called a 'slut')

- Understanding the impact of these dominant societal beliefs and how they might personally impact on our own sexual experiences can be key to changing our relationship with desire. This might include not feeling able to ask for what we like, feeling our pleasure is unimportant in comparison to someone else's, or being overly focused on the importance of how we look

Exercise:
Reflection: Your sexual biography

Reflect on your sexual history from as early in your life as you can remember and write a story of your emerging sexuality from:

- ➲ Your early memories of your body and self-touch and any reactions you remember the family having towards this

- ➲ How body parts were named when you were growing up

- ➲ Consent around your bodily autonomy

- ➲ Any unwanted sexual experiences, no matter how 'minor' you feel they were

- ➲ How your sexuality started to emerge with puberty, and the pride or shame you felt about this

- ➲ How sex was talked about, and what was implicit in those conversations

- ➲ How the significant adults in your life demonstrated their sexuality and what you took from this.

- ➲ How you have felt about your body since you were young. What can you remember thinking and feeling about your body, including body hair, your vulva, your weight, your breasts? What messages were around about what you 'should' look like?

- ➲ What was your experience of starting your periods, having early lustful feelings, your first sexual experiences and what part you learned to play in sex from an early age?

⮕ What you learned about what was important that you do or not do in sex, and why? Whose pleasure was prioritized, and how did you feel about this at the time?

⮕ Who did you talk to about masturbation? Sex?

⮕ What was the contribution of race, culture, ability, religion or age to this journey?

⮕ What were the messages you received from TV, magazines or porn, and how did this make a difference?

⮕ What messages about sex did you internalize that were entirely due to gender?

⮕ How did what you knew (or didn't know) about your own body make a difference to your sexual journey?

After you've written the story of your sexuality for yourself, think about:

1. The legacy of this story for any parts of your sex life in this present day (positive and negative)

2. Whether you continue to be influenced by ideas about sex or your body that you don't actually agree with and want to consciously try to move away from

3. Reflect on how you might do this. For example, are any of your current cultural and social contexts reinforcing these ideas? A good example of this is body image – it's rare to meet a woman who feels happy with her body or genitals when naked. This is mainly due to the constant barrage of media images representing 'perfect' bodies. A good way to start to tackle this is to change what you're exposed to – for example, by curating your social

media feeds. Being exposed to feeds with images of normal women, a variety of vulvas and body positivity will, over time, make a difference to how you feel about your own body

4. Being aware of these influences is one important step in taking away some of their power, but you can also make changes to the way that you act in relation to them. For example, if you have always believed that talking about sex is vulgar, talk about it more with friends or a partner. If you have always faked orgasms, see what happens if you don't. If you only ever have sex that ends with a penis in a vagina, experiment with changing this. At times, you may have to take yourself out of your comfort zone, but the impact of rejecting these scripts actively is key to changing the weight of their influence on your sex life

5

Sex in our relationships

'We want it to be like it was in the beginning'

In an era where lust and passion dominate our perspective of a good sexual connection and is often how a 'good sex life' is represented to us on screen, a sex life where passion can last the distance of time appears to be one of the holy grails of popular culture. In therapy sessions, I see many couples who come to see me because they want it 'to be like it was in the beginning'. Although sex therapy can create huge shifts in people's sex lives if people are committed to the process, it's often important to know that the feelings we might have in the early stages of a relationship – where we are driven to distraction by wanting, lust and obsessive thoughts – can't really last. Something else takes their place – an opportunity for knowing another person intimately (both physically, sexually and emotionally), and the foundations of a relationship (of whatever type and structure) that can lead to personal, sexual and emotional growth.

Is it possible to have good sex for ever?

It is absolutely possible to maintain high levels of sexual satisfaction and desire whilst having sex with the same person time and time again, but it requires some investment and, for most, some effort. The early stages of sexual relationships tend to be high in lust and

desire, and this time is characteristically different from more established stages of our sex lives, when we get to know our partners on a
deeper level. One of the great cruelties of this is that, for many
couples, the things that they value about a longer-term relationship
(security, knowing another person completely) can bring with them
an overfamiliarity and predictability that isn't always great for our
sex lives. If we add to this unhelpful and inaccurate societal messages that you should desire sex with a partner in a relationship often,
without having to do any work on triggering that desire, then we
can start to understand why sexual dissatisfaction within relationships
is a very common experience.

It might be obvious to state it, but sex happens in a context of other
relationship dynamics. This means that levels of contentment,
irritation, power play and connection/disconnection in the relationship influence how we feel we can be (and want to be) in relation to
sex. Sex with casual partners or even strangers is also not immune to
the impact of the relationship (even if it's a relationship of only an
hour) influencing how we act sexually – but there's an obvious
difference in us being less known to them and also knowing them
less. During sex we might find ourselves wanting to be passionate,
creative, assertive, subservient, quiet, aggressive, shy, serious, sensual,
dominant, playful – all kinds of things. For some of us, some of these
ways of expressing ourselves sexually are easier with a stranger,
as being a 'blank slate' in their eyes can allow us to feel less self-
conscious about showing a wider variety of these contrasting versions
of our sexual selves. We can feel freed from fearing that they will pick
up on this as unusual and say, 'Whoa! What's going on with you?
You're not usually like this!' This freedom can allow a greater variety
in expressing our sexual selves that, for some people, can feel
constraining in long-term relationships.

For others, taking a risk to show different sides of our sexual selves is easier to do in the safety and security of a relationship, where we feel safe to try new things, express ourselves fully and be totally free. At this point, it's worth considering your 'conditions for good sex' that you started to put together in Chapter 3. What kinds of ways of being do you have written down under psychological arousal? How many of these do you feel able to bring in to your sex life at the moment? Are there any types of sexual expression that feel out of bounds for whatever reason? Are there sides of your preferred sexual self, such as showing aggression or totally relinquishing control, that are easier with someone you trust or with a complete stranger?

I've met many people in my clinical work in long-term relationships who crave sex with a stranger, not entirely for the novelty of the stranger but for the novelty of being able to be a different person themselves. As well as the physical act of sex being vulnerable to becoming predictable over time, so can we as the players in that act. We risk becoming typecast, and the sides of ourselves that we show sexually can become narrow and predictable. Before we know it, we feel restricted in what parts we can play or who we can be, in a way that takes away variety in our expression of ourselves sexually.

Before Tom, Jess had enjoyed diversity in who she felt she was sexually and had enjoyed being both dominant and submissive in subtle ways, as well as having passionate sex, which felt frenzied, and sex which felt slow, intimate and sensual. When she met Tom, she enjoyed the fact that they had lots of intimate, sensual sex, and it fitted with the fact that she fell in love with him and the intensity of their emotional connection was high. Several years later, they were still in love, but Jess felt stifled by the dynamic between them sexually. It wasn't that she didn't enjoy the slow, sensual intimate sex that they had – she still did. But she missed a part of herself sexually that she had previously valued, the variety of expression that allowed sex, and crucially her own sexual expression, to be much more diverse.

You might be wondering what this has got to do with their relationship? After all, this is about Jess and what Jess wants, not Tom. But Jess sees herself and her way of being in the relationship through the lens of Tom's eyes. Their sexual personas have been defined by the sex they have been having and so Tom sees Jess as a sensual, intimate person sexually. Picking up on this, Jess feels self-conscious about acting outside of this role, so she does not try to show the sides of herself that she is finding herself missing. She also finds it hard to articulate the part that she'd quite like Tom to play sexually sometimes, which is to be assertive, dominant, selfish and impulsive. The limits that Tom and Jess's relationship dynamics place on their expression of sexuality place them at risk – not only of sexual boredom, but also of Jess feeling motivated to seek this interaction elsewhere. We're all capable of having non-negotiated sex outside of a monogamous relationship, for a huge variety of reasons, but sometimes these reasons are connected to parts of our sexuality that are stifled rather than our feelings about our sexual partners.

We shouldn't be fooled into thinking that monogamy is easy for most people, especially if we are clipping the wings of the full expression of our sexual personas or those of our partners, as it most definitely isn't. In fact, it has been suggested that it might be harder for women than for men, due to the impact of long-term monogamy on desire.[1] As the UK largely has been a monogamous society for the last few centuries (despite plenty of evidence that it doesn't work for many people), there is an assumption that mono-gamy is 'natural', easy, how humans work or without effort. This can be a dangerous place to be if we want to sustain mono-gamy, as it implies that monogamy will work for our relationship under any strain, circumstance or conditions. It also implies that there are people who are 'good and faithful' and people who are not, which is equally unhelpful. The truth is that choosing mono-gamy as a relationship structure might be just as 'challenging' as choosing a different relationship structure and should be approached as such.

It might be worth stopping here and reflecting on whether there are any sides of your sexual self that you'd like to show but currently feel restricted in showing or expressing. Fantasies are not necessarily indicative of what we want in real life, but there are some interest-ing parallels with how we see ourselves being in our fantasies (in control, passionate, devoured, taken, powerful) and what we might enjoy more of in our sexual expression in real life. Some fascinating research by Justin Lehmiller in 2018 into some of the most common fantasies and what they mean to people suggests that fantasies can be a window into our own sexual preferences when we don't feel restricted by what society dictates for our sex lives.[2]

Why does sex matter?

When a couple consults me around problems with desire, or fre-quency of sex in the relationship, it is *almost never* about the amount of desire or frequency of sex in the relationship. One of the tasks involved in making a meaningful change in the lives of a couple struggling with this is understanding what the real problem is.

What I mean by this is that the key to getting to the bottom of how we feel about our sex lives is understanding the meaning of sex for us as individuals, and for our relationships. Only then can we know what it is we feel we are missing out on if it's not happening as much as one or both of us would like, or in the way that we would like. Only once we know this can we understand the cost to that couple and why it might be troubling them right now. For Jess, her concerns about sex were that the relationship dynamic or sexual habits she and Tom had got into were, she felt, stifling her own sexual expression. But what beliefs and assumptions were behind how their sex life did or didn't play out?

When we talked further, it was clear that Tom's preference around how they had sex was not just about his 'conditions for good sex', but was connected to his perception of their relationship identity. Tom explained that he was desperately in love with Jess and that he wanted their sex life to represent that. Jess tentatively and nervously explained that sometimes she craved more 'animalistic sex' and had fantasies of being 'taken' by Tom in a way that was about his desire for her being about his physical wants, not their emotional connection. Tom was, at first, shocked and upset, as he felt this change signified a change in their relationship and one for the worse. He felt that the animalistic sex Jess was referring to represented a way men were with women when they were not respecting them. We talked more about it and started to understand this change in Jess's preference as being both about her wanting to revisit and express all sides of herself sexually, as she always had, as well as wanting some variety in the parts they played sexually, for the sake of novelty within their sex life. But we also understood it as being about the impact of having been together seven years, as Jess explained that she knew Tom loved her intensely, and she was very grateful for this, but that, after all this time, she craved feeling desired by him, and that this was one of the reasons this particular fantasy was a favourite of hers.

It's also important to notice here that Tom's assumption that sensual sex = love and animalistic sex = disrespect are an important aspect of the picture, as these societal and heavily gendered messages of how men should treat women influence the sex that Tom feels inclined to have. These beliefs might be Tom's individual 'conditions for good sex', but, for Tom (as with all of us), his conditions for good sex are heavily influenced by the role of society, gender politics and his learning about sex so far. It's interesting to note that it's also possible that there are sides of Tom's sexual self that he is restricting for fear of seeming disrespectful or trivializing their love, based on his assumptions about how sex should be, or his feminist views. Relationship dynamics, habits, communication and miscommunication are crucial to good sex, and are the focus of this chapter, but each person in the relationship brings with them their own beliefs, attitudes and past experience, which shapes the relationship dynamics. The interaction of the two plays out in the subtle and often unspoken dance between us.

For Jess and Tom, their sex life was hampered by the limitations, routine and habits their relationship had got into as these were restricting their sexual expression. This was heavily connected to the meanings they read into doing it differently. But the meanings we form about sex in our relationship are not always connected to how we or our partners are sexually, but sometimes more in relation to how much we want sex, or the importance we perceive our partners place on it.

Lucy was worried that Gina seemed to want sex much less now than she did when they first got together. She started to worry that this was about Gina not finding her attractive any more, but she didn't voice this concern outright, instead letting her dissatisfaction about their lack of sex come out in sarcastic comments during rows. Lucy was desperately worried about Gina no longer finding her attractive, as that was what had prompted the end of her last relationship and her confidence had been knocked so badly by it.

Lucy's concerns appear to be about the quantity of sex that they are having in their relationship, but there is a strong chance that this is just a surface-level concern. Lucy interpreted the change in frequency of sex as a signal that something else, something alarming, was wrong. For Lucy, Gina not wanting sex as much as she did signalled that she just wasn't good enough, wasn't attractive enough. Lucy internalized the problem as being about her (though, in actual fact, Gina had no idea Lucy had done this, as Gina was used to Lucy making jokes that *she* was the problem). For other people, differences in desire for sex can prompt fears of a fundamental lack of compatibility, and worries about the future of the relationship. Our individual beliefs about the meaning of sex are important in relationships, but we can also see the impact of beliefs about sex in society trickling down into our beliefs and creating a problem where there isn't necessarily one. Lucy was perhaps dialling into the strongly held societal belief that a woman's worth and sexual role are heavily based on her appearance, or maybe a fear about the myth of 'lesbian bed death'. Other beliefs affecting the personal meaning we make of a change in our sex lives can be 'you shouldn't have to work at sex, it just happens' and 'relationships must have a lot of sex to survive'. The impact of society, outlined in the previous chapter, is crucial here but, importantly, it's generally something in the relationship that has allowed this to take root and become a problem. It's likely that, if Lucy had voiced her concerns earlier, she may have got the reassurance she needed and the change in their sex life might not have felt like an issue. Talking about sex might sound easy but, as we all probably know, in reality it can feel like anything but.

Communication and initiation

Much has been written about the importance of communication for a good sex life. We know from research that people who are more able to talk about sex with partners enjoy their sex lives more,[3] and that communicating about sex acts as a buffer to a drop in desire.[4] This includes being able to talk about what you like, don't like, your fantasies and desires, and your evolving wants, need and preferences. Sounds simple, right? Well, it might be if we didn't have all the gaps in our foundations that we talked about in Chapter 2. Being out of practice, not having the right words, feeling shame or being raised with the belief that talking about sex is crass can all get in the way. Getting the words out can make us feel incredibly vulnerable and anxious – I see this all the time in sex therapy, even in the most confident and outspoken of people. No matter how good we are at talking generally, we're all still up against it, as we live in a world where it's not okay to talk about sex.

This matters for several reasons. Firstly, because our sexuality (our wants, needs and preferences) changes over our lifetime, and we and our partners need to be able to know about and talk about this, so that we can adapt to it. For example, 'Since I've been pregnant, I actually really like penetrative sex in a way I wasn't that fussed about before, can we start doing more of it?'

Secondly, the very nature of sex is negotiation. On a broad level this might be 'what kind of sex life do we want to have as a couple?'; week by week it might be 'I want sex now, do you?'; and, in the moment, negotiations like 'I want to do X to you but I'm not sure if you want that or not.' Negotiation is difficult without communication. Imagine trying to get anything else in life done in partnership with someone else without being able to talk about it? Talking about sex is essential for negotiation, and negotiation is crucial to good sex. At the start of a relationship, or when things are going well, it may appear that sex just happens and doesn't need negotiation. This is not strictly true, but it can be more easily masked during this early stage, when desire and lust are high. But the challenge comes when we want something different, when problems crop up or when life gets in the way. By then we can be out of practice with negotiating about sex, but getting back into practice can be especially hard if we find talking and listening to each other already challenging, even outside of sex. It can also be difficult if we have both grown a little defensive about our sexual relationship or generally find it hard to assert our wants and needs.

Lastly, communication in sex is important because we are heavily influenced by the world we live in and, unless we are able to explicitly state otherwise, we risk being shoehorned into a model of what society tells us sex *should* be like. This can be what we think we should be doing based on sexual scripts rather than what we *actually want*. For example, we might need to actively say, 'I actually could take or leave penetrative sex, to be honest. Can we not always do it? In fact, I'd be happy if only 10% of our sex ended this way,' or else penetrative sex will be assumed to be our main event and this will affect our satisfaction and desire in the long term if it's not our favourite thing.

I could share a million examples with you from the couples I've worked with. Everything from difficulty in asking to use lube ('they'll see it as a sign that I'm not turned on enough'), to asking for oral sex ('I'm pretty sure he doesn't like it as he doesn't often do it') to how sex is initiated ('she thinks I like it when she bites my ear but I find it cringey'). Quite often one of the key turning points in therapy comes when something that has never previously been spoken about is talked about in detail, and we discover that neither person was right about what they thought the other person thought about it. In therapy, sometimes we call this 'the difference which makes a difference' (a phrase coined by systemic therapist Gregory Bateson).[5] These turning points in therapy demonstrate the power of 'not talking' in keeping us stuck in old patterns that are not helpful. Sex, in my opinion, is the area of our lives and relationships which is most ripe for miscommunication. To keep sex good and to benefit our desire in the long term, talking about sex is crucial.

As I mentioned earlier, it sounds simple, but we all know that being socialized not to talk about it, not having the words for it or not feeling comfortable saying the words out loud can make it hard. Imagine trying to order some new books you've been wanting to read in a bookshop that you've been raised to feel ashamed to shop in. The titles of the books you want contain words you've never spoken out loud before and also words you associate with embarrassment. There's the added impact of being socialized to feel shame about ordering these books, as people might take one look at you and expect you to want totally different books (or no books at all).

In some ways, when I'm doing sex therapy, I'm the person working in the bookshop. I try to make customers feel that it's perfectly okay for them to be shopping here, or to help out by first offering a few titles of books they might be interested in, without any prejudice about what they might like (also, being the first person to say the words can be hard, so it's easier if I start things off). I might make some suggestions for good titles if they're really struggling, encouraging them to try not to be influenced by what they think others might read. Even with someone facilitating, talking about sex can be hard, but without good communication our sex lives and our desire will suffer.

You will know yourself how easy or difficult you find talking about *anything* tricky generally in your relationship, and this might be a good barometer for considering how communication might be helping or hindering your sex life, given sex is usually harder to discuss than most things. How well do you feel you and your partner currently communicate? Do you feel listened to? Taken seriously? Are difficult topics easy or hard to bring up? Do they get quickly sidelined when they get tough, or can you both stick with it and find a way to delve in even if it's uncomfortable? Does one of you use humour in a way that the other finds dismissive? Does one of you wish the other would use humour a bit more to lighten the tone? Does one (or both) of you interpret any difficult conversation as criticism, or feel frightened and get defensive? Do you feel able to take responsibility for whatever you are talking about in equal measure, or does one of you always seem to bear the brunt of blame? Do you struggle not to be 'right', are you both able to really, intently listen and hear not just the words but the feelings behind them? Are you able to admit you were wrong and say sorry?

There's plenty of help out there for improving your communication as a couple generally, and if reading this segment has got you thinking that you could do with making some changes in this regard, I'd recommend you first find a way to work on communication outside of your sex life, so that the changes you make benefit what happens inside your sex life too. Later on, in Part Three, we'll revisit the idea of how to talk about making changes in your sex life in a way that works, and I'll be recommending some strategies on how to do this. These strategies will be useful only if there aren't fundamental issues in your communication already that could do with addressing, however, so take action now if needed.

Of course, we could be forgiven for thinking that communication about sex is mainly talking about it. In fact, there is a whole host of complex non-verbal or indirect communications that we use to communicate in the absence of, or in addition to, words, and these can be just as useful and just as problematic. Take Axa and Jack as an example:

Axa had been thinking about Jack during the day at work and was generally feeling content and lucky to be in a relationship with him. She decided it would be great to have sex tonight, mainly as she wanted to demonstrate her love to him, but also as it made her feel on cloud nine to connect with him that way. Axa sends a text to Jack saying, 'Let's have a cosy night in tonight ☺', hoping that Jack will understand what she means. When they get home, Axa dresses in an outfit she knows Jack likes and puts some music on that she finds sensual. Jack comes in and is clearly pleased to see her, but seems distracted about his day and the relentless sound of an album he finds annoying. They sit on the sofa together, and Axa asks about his day, all the while stroking the back of his neck with her fingers and looking him in the eye. She kisses him, and he kisses back but pulls away to tell her about another thing that happened which he forgot to mention. Axa asks him if he wants dinner, or to take a bath together. He replies that he's quite hungry, so dinner would be good. When it's time for bed, Axa takes off her clothes in front of Jack, looks him straight in the eye and places his hand on her naked body. She sees the glimmer of recognition in his face.

How many indirect or non-verbal communications did you notice Axa making before Jack understood what she was getting at? We might call this initiation. Initiation of sex (and by 'sex', I of course mean any sexual act) is simply a communication that says, 'shall we . . . ?' It can be tricky, particularly as it can be direct ('I'm horny and I'd like to go down on you? Can I?') or indirect, such as the strategies Axa tries above. Initiation is an important part of sex with someone else, but it also depends, crucially, on communication and, as with any communication, it's ripe for misunderstanding and misinterpretation. This is something that many couples struggle with. One person has the thought or motivation to be sexual, but the other doesn't notice the initiation as the communication is too indirect, or they have misinterpreted it as non-sexual, or it comes at a time when they are too absorbed in something else. The opposite can also happen – our sexual communication can feel blunt and too much for our partner, and they experience it as pressure to feel something that they currently don't. More about how initiation fits in with desire and an opportunity to spot how this happens in your own relationships, helping or hindering desire, can be found in Chapter 7.

In the meantime, a few fascinating facts about initiation of sex: it's heavily linked with sexual scripts, and research over the last few decades has shown that women in relationships with men are initiating sex more than they used to, reflecting a change in the (outdated but still somewhat influential) scripts that 'men should initiate sex more than women' and 'men are the drivers and women are the gatekeepers of sex'. This is a positive change for women's sexuality, as we know that being the person who initiates sex is also associated with higher levels of sexual satisfaction in the sexual encounter that follows.

Although women in relationships with men initiate sex roughly equally as often as men, research tells us that they tend to initiate sex more directly than men.[6] This means that women in relationships with men are more likely to say, 'I'm feeling horny, let's have sex' than to start kissing a partner gently and hope they know what this means. There have been some ideas put forward as to why this is the case, especially given that we know women who have sex with women (who, incidentally, report initiating sex more than women in relationships with men) tend to use more indirect strategies. Sex researchers suggest that the script that 'men are always up for sex' (which, as you now know, is also not true) is still very much alive and kicking, and responsible for women who have sex with men feeling more able to take a risk with direct communication. In contrast, women who have sex with other women, and men having sex with women, might do the opposite and assume that women are more likely not to feel like sex, and so 'test the waters' of initiation more gently.

A final word on initiation. It's normal and common to often not feel like sex at the same time as someone else, but how we convey that to a partner can have an important consequence on our sexual satisfaction long term. For example, research tells us that 'rejecting' a partner in a reassuring way ('I'd really like to and I am really attracted to you but I just have all this work to do') leads to higher levels of couple satisfaction long term than a critical way ('Why are you so sex mad all the time? I wish you'd stop nagging me about it.)[7]

Why we have sex

Why is sex important to us, our partners and our relationship and why does it matter if we don't have it? Well, partly, the answer to this is linked with the reasons we have sex in the first place. Representations in the media will have you believe that sexual activity happens as a response to feeling sexual desire, but, that is not necessarily the case, especially in a long-term relationship. Of course we want arousal and desire to be present at some point in the sexual encounter, and sex will be pretty rubbish without it making an appearance, but it's often not there in the beginning – it grows over time, so there's another need being met at the beginning that it's important we are paying attention to. It's these needs which, without sex, we or our partners feel we are missing out on and can cause us distress.

In 2007 sex researchers Cindy Meston and David Buss did some research into the reasons people engaged in sex. Before their study, a few other studies had reported a handful of motivations, such as 'I felt horny', 'to relieve sexual tension' or 'to be emotionally close'. Meston and Buss found there was much more to it than this – 237 distinct reasons, in fact, linked with other aspects of psychological functioning, whether it was with casual, regular or relationship partners.[8] Gender played a big part in the reported reasons, with some themes of emotion as a driver rated highly for women and physical sensation rated highly for men. This is unsurprising, due to the social conditioning of how messages around gender play into our learning about sex over the years.

Some of these needs or motivations relate to pleasure, some to protecting the relationship, some to expressing or feeling attractive; some are about placating and some are about obligation, boredom, stress relief or self-expression. Take a minute to consider how these drivers or motivations are represented in society and the media. Sexual desire is almost always portrayed as uncontainable passion or lust. We rarely see representations of sex that start as one person going along with another's initiation but end up being passionate and hot, but this is a lived experience for many people and is perfectly good sex. What I'd like you to take away from this is that the desperate I-want-to-tear-your-clothes-off-now desire is not always the driver for many people. It is also not very realistic in long-term relationships.

Sometimes not having sex or not having enough sex is what is named as a problem by one or both people. However, in my experience, after some detailed enquiry into this, people will say that, actually, there's something else behind this that's bothering them. Things like the conflict it causes, feeling abnormal, worrying about infidelity as a result of not 'satisfying' their partner, feeling rejected, missing the excitement it brings, missing expressing that part of themselves, feeling disconnected, etc., etc.

What this means is that concerns about what is happening in your sex life might not necessarily be linked with how much sex you are having, but rather that one or both of you are losing the opportunity to meet other needs in that particular way. A sexual partner will have their own key drivers or motivations for sex, things they really value, reasons why they are inclined to want sex. Do you know what they are? How do we know why they feel the way they do about the amount or type of sex you are currently having if we do not know what function sex serves for them?

Understanding this about ourselves and our relationships can be the first step in getting to the bottom of the problem of what's missing for us and our partners when we're not having the greatest sexual connection or experiencing a discrepancy in desire (both of which are inevitable for all of us, at times). Understanding this also gives us some useful clues about how we can address these needs in other ways – either while we work on sex, instead of sex or in addition to it.

Let's go back to Axa and Jack for a second. Re-read this description of them from earlier, and see what you make of Axa's motivations to initiate being sexual with Jack.

Axa had been thinking about Jack during the day at work and was generally feeling content and lucky to be in a relationship with him. She decided it would be great to have sex tonight, mainly as she wanted to demonstrate her love to him, but also as it made her feel on cloud nine to connect with him that way. Axa sends a text to Jack saying, 'Let's have a cosy night in tonight ☺', hoping that Jack will understand what she means. When they get home, Axa dresses in an outfit she knows Jack likes and puts some music on that she finds sensual. Jack comes in and is clearly pleased to see her, but seems distracted about his day and the relentless sound of an album he finds annoying. They sit on the sofa together, and Axa asks about his day, all the while stroking the back of his neck with her fingers and looking him in the eye. She kisses him, and he kisses back but pulls away to tell her about another thing that happened that he forgot to mention. Axa asks him if he wants dinner, or to take a bath together. He replies that he's quite hungry, so dinner would be good. When it's time for bed, Axa takes off her clothes in front of Jack, looks him straight in the eye and places his hand on her naked body. She sees the glimmer of recognition in his face.

What did you notice?

Axa is not feeling desire. Axa is wanting to have sex because it meets her need to express her love for Jack, allowing her to feel close and connected with him. This is an important difference. If Jack had decided that he didn't want to be sexual with Axa this evening, the consequence for Axa is not one of sexual frustration, but of missing out on an opportunity to connect and show love for Jack. This motivation can be met in ways other than sex, but if neither Axa nor Jack recognizes that this is what Axa is wanting, the sex (or lack of it) might be incorrectly assumed to be the problem between them. Sex may well be the vehicle for another need.

There are many reasons why understanding your and your partner's motivations for sex are important. An easy trap to fall into if your partner is the one who initiates sex more than you is to assume that their initiation is solely motivated by a need to release sexual tension, or to express a 'sex drive' unconnected to you. This might well be the case (and certainly will be for all of us on certain occasions), but this is where some of our sexual scripts can trip us up. If you're trying to negotiate a difference in desire with a male partner, scripts that 'men always want sex' and talk of men thinking of sex every seven seconds can reduce the entirety of men's sexual behaviour to nothing more than scratching an itch. The truth is that men are much more complex, as are women. We all have complex reasons for wanting sex, which if we were more aware of, might lead us to be more empathetic when we are turning each other down, or to find other ways to meet that need.

Since Meston and Buss's original research into people's motivations to be sexual, other researchers have started to investigate whether the *type of motivation* a person has for having sex matters.[9] They investigated what difference it made to people's sex lives when they were motivated to have sex by a positive outcome, such as giving or receiving pleasure or to experience intimacy (termed 'approach' reasons), as compared to those who were motivated to have sex to avoid negative outcomes, such as conflict, a partner's disappointment, or to prevent a partner leaving (termed 'avoidance' reasons). The results were fascinating. It turns out that having sex for avoidance reasons is more likely to result in a decline in sexual satisfaction over time. On the other hand, having sex for approach reasons is associated with increased sexual satisfaction as well as the person holding a more positive view of sex. What's useful to know from a desire perspective is that not only is having sex for approach reasons associated with better sex, but it has also been shown to buffer against sexual desire dropping over time.[10]

In my work I often meet couples who are having sex because one person wants to (and is annoyed if they don't 'get it') and another person is feeling little desire to but is having sex to 'keep the peace'. This is likely to further reduce desire over time for the person going along with it. In addition to this, this same crucial research into the impact of approach or avoidance reasons on a partner has found that, despite people often having this type of avoidance sex to please a partner, it doesn't actually achieve this result, as sexual partners of people having sex for avoidance goals report less satisfaction also. What this means is that it might feel like it's helping to have sex to placate someone else, but it is not actually helping anyone. Instead, it's possibly making the situation worse over time for both of you. If this is the case for you, then it is important to address it by stopping having sex for these reasons. Instead, studies have shown that if you ask people to focus more on approach reasons (for example, thinking about and noting down positive reasons why they might want to be sexual), they experience higher levels of sexual satisfaction and desire than people who have not been instructed to do this.[11] This is a wonderful piece of sex science, as it shows us that we can modify our motivations (and therefore our satisfaction and desire) simply by intentionally focusing on all the good things that we or our relationships stand to gain from sex.

At the end of this chapter you'll find a more detailed exercise to help you consider your motivations for yourself and encourage your partner to do so also. You can then start to consider the pattern of this in your relationship and work out what function sex serves for the two of you. Is it mainly to connect? Is it to feel and express attraction? Is it to experience another level of sensation/experience together that marks you out as a sexual couple? Is it to keep each other satisfied as a strategy to protect the relationship from infidelity? Is it to escape from the mundane and feel alive? Are your motivations for sex largely approach or avoidance based? Once you have done this, I'd like you to use this information to reduce or stop having sex for avoidance reasons (explaining to your partner why this is important, as well as understanding what their motivations are and how they can be met in other ways) in addition to spending more time investing in and thinking about approach goals.

Whatever the function that sex serves for you, your partner and the relationship, understanding this allows the two of you to know what difference it would make if you invested in it more, what you stand to lose if you don't and how your motivations might affect your desire over time.

Desire discrepancy between people in a relationship

In Chapter 3 we talked about data from the most recent Natsal study, which told us that about a quarter of UK adults feel like they have a different level of desire to their partner. So the issue of trying to negotiate a difference in desire is not solely the problem of couples seeking sex therapy, but rather an experience common to many of us, and it is likely to be a challenge that most of us will need to negotiate in our sex lives. The problem comes when we don't know how to manage this difference between us, or when it starts to feel loaded, hurtful or frustrating. How it feels when we feel like having sex less frequently than our partner depends on the meaning we make of sex, and why it's important to us. So let's try to understand this in a little more detail.

One of the first things I do when a couple comes to see me, telling me that one of them has 'low sexual desire' that is causing them both distress, is to explain to couples that I prefer to talk about it not as one person's problem with *low desire*, but as a problem of *discrepancy of desire* in their relationship, which is standing in the way of one (or both) of them getting something they need. Or I might explain it as a problem of a mismatch between how they feel and an unrealistic standard set for them by society around the myth of spontaneous sexual desire for women in their long-term relationship. Or that it's a problem of how the comfort or pattern of their relationship over time has unwittingly turned into a barrier to desire flourishing. This subtle change in seeing a problem of desire as *not one person's problem* and using language which shows that it's dependent on other things and amenable to change is where the hope builds (and the work starts).

Relationship dynamics and sex

The impact that relationships with significant people, such as early caregivers, have on our lives is known as our 'attachment style'. Attachment theory, initially reported by the child psychoanalyst John Bowlby, is a way of acknowledging that humans have a natural propensity to seek out closeness with others, and that our ability to trust and feel secure with another person or feel loved is something we learn from the world around us in the first few years of life. This learning happens through our interactions with our attachment figures, who, when we are babies and young children, are our primary caregivers. We can develop a 'secure attachment style' when we feel that we are (more often than not) responded to, our needs are met and our caregiver is available and responsive. This leads us to develop a positive sense of ourselves and others that we take with us throughout life, influencing our expectations (and therefore our behaviour) in all future relationships.

On the other hand, if we experience our caregiver as mostly rejecting, unavailable or to be feared, we can develop an 'anxious' or 'avoidant' attachment style. This means that our early learning is that other people cannot be trusted, don't meet our needs, or will not come back when we need them. Again, this will influence our relationships as we move through life, leading us to be hypervigilant to rejection, or fearful or uncomfortable getting close to, or relying on others.

In adulthood our attachment figures are typically the people or person we reach out to if we are upset, or need care or support, which is often a romantic/sexual partner. It's good to know that even if we've had a difficult early start and developed an anxious attachment style (for example, being prone to regular fear that our partner will leave, and showing a lot of hypervigilance or reassurance seeking around this), our attachment style can change with new experiences of someone who offers security. This means that, if someone who has an anxious attachment style is with someone who is consistently reassuring and dependable, a more secure attachment can emerge, and worry about being abandoned can start to diminish.

The interaction between our attachment style and that of our partner is relevant to desire and the approach / avoidance motivations for sex we covered a few pages ago. For example, it can be harder not to have sex for avoidance reasons (i.e. to prevent a partner from leaving you for not 'giving them sex') if you are someone who finds it difficult to trust that people will stay, or that you are worthy of people staying.[12] This can make it challenging not to have sex for avoidance reasons, and, in this case, it's useful to consider how you can start to feel more secure in the relationship, so that you can feel confident in asserting yourself in this way now you know the effect that sex for avoidance reasons could have on desire.

For some people, therapy can be a useful way of figuring out whether they have a way of relating to others that's affecting their sex life problematically in the here and now. Not everyone needs therapy, however, and for some people, understanding what's going on in their sex life in this way (by questioning the function sex serves and whether their reasons are approach or avoidance), in combination with having a reassuring partner, can be a way of bringing added security to the picture.

Bad sex equals bad relationship, right?

No, not necessarily. It can be easy to assume that, if things aren't working perfectly when it comes to sex, there must be something wrong, but it's often not the case. It's certainly true that there's a direct relationship between how content we are in our relationship and our sexual satisfaction, and how content we are with our sexual relationship and relationship satisfaction, and it's perhaps common sense to recognize why. But it doesn't follow like this for all couples. For some couples, the relationship couldn't be any better, but good sex, or even any sex, feels hard to achieve. This can happen for so many reasons, but can include things like getting out of the habit of relating to each other sexually and starting to feel more like friends than partners, waiting for desire to come spontaneously but not creating the context for it, or being so intimate that it's hard to position the other as sexual. So let's discuss some of the relationship dynamics or habits we can fall into which might get in the way of desire, even in the most solid relationship.

Intimacy – too little or too much?

Intimacy (which may mean something different to you than to the next person) is also an interesting concept when it comes to the success of a sexual relationship. When people use the word 'intimacy' they often mean emotional closeness or connection, trust, security or familiarity. This might show itself in everything from how much time they spend apart, how much they share of their personal thoughts and feelings, or the personal boundaries they feel comfortable to cross, such as how comfortable they feel about going to the toilet in front of each other. There are no rights or wrongs when it comes to levels of intimacy, in that we all have our own preferences regarding what feels good to us, and what works. But despite much advice around spending more time together or ramping up intimacy being good for your sex life, it's possible that this is not always the best advice, at least not for all couples. There are certainly some relationships where an increase in intimacy could lead to a better sexual connection, perhaps as it brings with it an opportunity to really connect, to feel safe, or to trust enough to let go of inhibitions. For other relationships, intimacy can do the opposite. Intimacy that prevents individuality, space, time to yearn for the other, the opportunity to see the other person as separate from yourself, or enough difference to create a feeling of novelty can be challenging for desire,[13] and having distance from a partner can buffer against this.[14] One of the things I'm often looking for when a couple first meets with me is how much physical separation there is between them, and how this helps or hinders their relationship. Only you will know whether intimacy is something you might benefit from fostering, or whether you might benefit from more distance in a metaphorical rather than a literal sense. There is also evidence that creating *changes in intimacy* is more important in boosting desire than striving for either extreme.[15] If you're interested in seeing the difference this may make in your relationship, perhaps experimenting by trying things differently for a few weeks might give you the information you need.

The paradox of security

'We do not own our partner. At best they are on loan to us, with a chance to renew.'

The above quote from Esther Perel (who has written extensively and eloquently about relationship dynamics, intimacy and desire)[16] is a wondrous challenge to our tendency to feel that our relationship and our partners are a given. It's provocative, as it is at odds with our societal expectations of monogamy as something that is easy and expected, as outlined in the previous chapter. It suggests that our partner could leave us at any time and that we should treat them and the relationship as if this were the case. How does reading this quote make you feel? Worried? Shocked? There are some remarkable benefits that can come of treating your relationship, no matter how long it has stood the test of time, as if it's something delicate and precious that needs to be nurtured to survive. I'm not suggesting for a second that we should not plan that cinema night out next week, or that holiday in three months, for fear that our partner might get up and leave tomorrow. But rather, if we take them too much for granted, due to a (mistaken) belief in the infallibility of monogamy or the institute of marriage, we might not see how crucial it is to nurture them and the relationship.

In therapy, I sometimes talk about the concept of what I call 'giving each other the scraps'. This is a relationship habit that can be easy to fall into, and is basically when we present the most exciting, dynamic, interested, interesting, attentive and caring sides of ourselves to our job, our friends, our work colleagues, our neighbours (or even the barista at Pret), but when we get home and see our partners we give one-word answers, lie on the sofa and barely make eye contact. Giving each other the scraps could also be positively construed as the joy of having a committed other who you don't always have to be presenting the best version of yourself to, someone you can completely relax around and just 'be'. This in itself is a wonderful thing. But there's also a risk that you and your partner could start to forget those sides of each other (that were so present and abundant in the early days) of making each other laugh, really listening to each other like no one else matters, of connecting over your hopes, dreams, knowledge and world view. This is where desire can suffer.

It's not the time you have but what you do with it that counts

A recent paper by Dr Amy Muise and her colleagues in Canada has added to what we know about how we spend time with our partners and the impact of this on sex.[17] We already know that couples who engage in activities that excite and inspire them with a partner revisit some of those much sought-after early relationship feelings towards one another, and Muise and her colleagues wanted to look at the impact of these same behaviours on sexual desire. Their recently published study suggests that an injection of novelty and 'self-expansion' in ourselves or our relationship outside the bedroom can affect what happens within it, and that couples who spend more time doing novel, interesting and challenging activities individually or together see an improvement in their sex life as a result. Self-expansion might include learning a new language, visiting a new place, taking on a physical challenge, or having a new experience.

Basically, they found that couples who spent time on these 'self-expansion' activities (as opposed to just time together as usual) were more likely to experience sexual desire, and more likely to have sex. What's important here is that it was not the amount of time couples spent together but how they spent it that resulted in higher reported desire and sexual activity. Couples who found ways to 'excite, inspire and connect' with each other in this way are thought to make space to learn new things about themselves or each other, and create conditions of novelty, distance and newness, akin to those in the early months and years together, fanning the flames of desire. A crucial finding of this study was that the longer sexual partners had been together, or the more pressed for time they were (think new parents), the more impact self-expansion activities such as these had on their sex lives. Our experiences of desire and sexual satisfaction are complex and there are many elements adding to this picture (what's going on in our bodies, our personal relationship with sex, our relationship with our cultural and social contexts), but there is a huge and tangible real-life value in studies such as this, which demystify how nurturing the seemingly non-sexual parts of our relationships can make a difference.

For our long-term sexual relationships, this means that, if we want to keep our sex lives hot, perhaps it's time to prioritize making time to really connect, by having explorative and meaningful conversations with the intention of discovering new things about each other – not just about what we ate for lunch or who said what at the photocopier. For some of us it might be as simple as looking at each other through another person's eyes, or in a different environment, such as watching our partners charm the new neighbours at a party. For others it might be planning an adventure together, trying something new and exhilarating, or learning how to dance. The bottom line is: the challenge of creating time together which involves something novel and exciting might take a bit of thought and planning, but it could seriously benefit our sex lives.

Consider some of these ideas around relationship dynamics and sex in your own life for a second. Do you feel that you spend so much time together that you know what your partner is about to say even before they do? Do you notice that you feel more desire when you've spent time apart? Do you feel that the more time you spend together, the more emotionally connected and sexual you feel? Do you sometimes wish you could live a more separate life and develop more of your own separate interests? Can you remember the last time you really laughed, felt excited or exhilarated together?

You probably have a natural reaction to reading this and know instinctively what camp you fall into. Would your relationship benefit from more or less emotional intimacy? Would it benefit from less time together, but for more of the time you spend together to be not just giving each other the scraps? Perhaps you don't feel that emotionally connected at all, and more time investing in your relationship is what's needed. Whichever it is, don't be fooled into thinking that spending time in the same room, house or flat constitutes this time. The opposite of giving each other the scraps is what's needed. Really connecting, listening and valuing each other's thoughts or opinions, without your TV or phone competing for your attention, is key. It's great to do this over dinner, or whenever you see each other, but if you can find time for self-expanding activities, such as doing something new together, having an adventure or engaging in a fun task together, then this kind of time together is probably the best type of all.

Priorities, practicalities and time together

In the last chapter we talked about the sexual script that 'sex should happen spontaneously and easily, without effort'. In my opinion, this is one of the fundamental challenges to good sex within modern-day relationships. We live in a society where we are told that to have a healthy body we must pay attention to our diet, to be fit and strong we must make time for a regular exercise routine, and to be happy we must find time to practise self-care and gratitude. It is less common to hear about the importance of prioritizing our sex life, or the benefits of doing so in this way. It's also common for practicalities and time together to be a bigger problem for desire than anything else, such as in the case of Alexandra and Gregory.

Alexandra and Gregory came to see me about the lack of sex in their relationship of three years. They explained that they wanted to have more of a sex life, but since about eight months after they'd been together, the frequency of sex between them had dwindled to once every month or two. Neither of them felt happy with this arrangement and both felt they were missing out on a connection unique to them, and feared what they had was turning into a sexless relationship, which would make their relationship more vulnerable to failure [hopefully you can spot here their motivations for sex, the function sex serves in their relationship, as well as the influence of societal beliefs and how crucial these are]. Once we'd established why this was important to them, and that there were clear benefits in making changes (instead of just accepting that once every two months was fine for them), we set to work on understanding how sex happened in their relationship. One of the key factors, they explained, was that they had no time for sex. I asked more about their commitments in other areas of their life and how they spent their time and they told me that they were on special diets to maintain their physiques, which required several hours of menu planning, shopping and meal prep every day. It became clear that it was not the case that they did not have time for sex, but rather that they did not prioritise sex in the way that they prioritized other elements of their life (their diet and fitness, which they put tremendous effort into). We wondered together what difference it would make if they spent several hours a day prioritizing their emotional and physical connection. I asked them, 'What if sex had the same priority as your diet?'.

Alexandra and Gregory admitted that they had never considered that they needed to prioritize sex before, as they thought it should just happen. But when they actually looked at their week and thought about it, there was not a single bit of free time or an obvious time of the day or week that gave them an opportunity to be sexual together. Understanding this meant that they then had two choices moving forward. The first was recognizing that sex is not happening as it's not a priority and changing the meaning of it so it's no longer seen as a problem ('We are not broken sexually. It's just that sex doesn't often happen spontaneously when you're busy doing other things and we have other priorities that are currently more important to us, and that is fine.'). The other choice is to decide what priority they want sex to take and treat it accordingly. This might mean relegating something else and making sacrifices in other areas, to devote the time to sex that it needs.

Even if it were true that sex happens spontaneously and easily without effort (which it mostly isn't), how would this spontaneity and ease happen if you aren't physically in the same room alone together? Think about your week with your partner for a second. Discount any time that you have with kids, family or other people in close proximity, discount any time you are at work, exercising or seeing friends. Discount any time you are getting dressed, cooking, cleaning or doing essential life admin. Discount the time you are asleep. How much time is left? By the time you've totted it all up, you might feel like all you want to do is watch Netflix and scroll through Instagram. You'd be normal in this regard. But if this is the case, how much of a challenge is it to expect sex to happen spontaneously and easily in this narrow window? Then add into the mix the need for your partner to be on the same page in terms of also feeling like sex spontaneously at exactly the same moment and we start to see what a challenge this is.

So what do you do if you only have late evenings alone together? What do you do if you feel most receptive to sex in the early morning, when things are hectic and you're both always rushing? Or perhaps in the middle of the day, when you are at work? What if you and your partner are on completely different time clocks with sex and you have a huge daily 'to do' list? This will undoubtedly affect your desire and is really common. In this case (and like Alexandra and Gregory), you have two options. One is to find more time together, that's uninterrupted and about connection on an emotional and physical level. The second is to change the meaning of what's happening with sex to be about the stage or pace of your lives rather than a problem between you. This might be enough to make it acceptable, or it might be that a sacrifice is needed. That's for you to decide.

For us to improve our sexual lives or keep them good over time, we must find a way for sex to feature in our priority list, or else we risk it becoming extinct. As much as we might not want to hear it, we have a choice in how we spend our (potentially small amount of) free time, but the choices we make inevitably side-line one activity over another (Netflix vs Sex) or by nature of how these impact our mood and therefore also impact on sex. For example, if we scroll social media and see a range of pictures and posts that make us feel low and feel self-critical, as opposed to spending time talking about our day whilst looking into our partner's eyes, leading to an increase in emotional intimacy. It might sound obvious when presented this way, but we don't always make the choices that match up best to our life or relationship goals.

Technology and our sex lives

Whilst we're on the subject of scrolling, smartphones are not always the greatest thing for sex when it comes to how we prioritize our time. Large-scale research studies both in the UK and the US has shown that couples are having less sex than ever before, and we can only guess that the key factor that has changed in the last ten years is the rise in smartphones to manage our day-to-day lives. The average Brit checks their phone every twelve minutes and spends about three hours a day using it to go online for things like social media, surfing the web or checking emails.[18] We look them more in the eye than we do our partners.

Our phones can sometimes take us away from the people we are with, into another world. They can also add another element of a life task into our day, as we feel the need to answer those work emails at home or catch up on Twitter, Facebook and Instagram every day. How much time do they take out of your day? Getting used to a constant level of stimulation from scrolling social media, watching TV and streaming online doesn't just take up a great deal of our time which we could be using to connect with others, though; they also make it harder for us to tolerate just being in the moment without being stimulated by them (how long can you sit in a restaurant when the person has gone to the toilet without getting out your phone?). Have a think about whether the time you spend on your phone or the power it has to distract you takes you away from your partner.

Of course, it's not technology per se that can have a negative impact on our sex lives, but the way in which we relate to it. Spending an hour a day on WhatsApp might be great for you if you're spending it flirting and sending images and promises of things to come. Scrolling Instagram for three hours per week, however, might be sapping time you could devote to emotionally connecting with your partner, or it could be your way of connecting with your sexuality, or working on your body positivity, by interacting with accounts focused on sex-positive messages, erotica, or images of body diversity. Technology isn't the problem, but not spending time reflecting on how it is helping or hindering your sex life might be.

Having children

There are a multitude of ways in which having a family can impact on our or our partner's desire for sex. On a biological level, breast-feeding can reduce desire due to the impact of the rise in the desire-sapping hormone prolactin, as can recovery from birth or the effects of birth trauma. But one of the biological factors that is perhaps most long-lasting after the birth is sleep deprivation. Whether you have children or not (but it will be ten times more applicable to you if you do), tiredness is a well-known desire killer. In fact, tired-ness is so influential for all of us in terms of our sex life that one study into women's desire, orgasm and arousal showed that getting enough sleep increases your chances of having sex the next day by 14%![19]

There's a well-documented and significant negative impact that having children has on our sex lives. Studies into the sex lives of new parents make for fairly depressing reading, mainly as sex tends to take such a hit in the first five years of having kids, and this can show itself in dissatisfaction or sexual problems at higher levels than those of the general population.[20] The important thing here is that it's not kids per se that impact on our sex lives and desire, but the changes that they bring with them. Having little people manhandling your body all the time or the loss of time to invest in activities that previously may have increased our confidence, desire or a sense of connection with our partner is the issue. Changes to our bodies post pregnancy, affecting body confidence, or an increased life admin or stress impacting on relationship dynamics are a factor too, as in the case of Sandra and Mike.

Having kids and the maternity leave that followed had kick-started more of a 'traditional' family structure, in terms of gender roles, than Sandra and Mike had ever intended, but they had become entrenched in these roles over the years. Sandra, previously attracted to Mike for his independence and egalitarian attitude towards their relationship, had started to be resentful of having taken over all of the responsibility for the household since going on maternity leave. She not only felt less desire for Mike as a result of this, but the position she found herself in of cooking, cleaning and making Mike's packed lunches was also a role she found deeply unsexy. At first Mike didn't understand how this could be influencing Sandra's desire for sex, mainly as he believed that sex was a drive that should happen spontaneously, regardless of what was going on in their lives.

In part, this is why not understanding how desire works can stop us finding solutions. Sandra and Mike are not alone in this aspect of the practical side of their relationship, i.e. division of labour impacting on their sex life. Studies have found that the more equitable the division of household tasks in relationships, the greater relationship and sexual satisfaction the couple usually report.[21] Sadly, even in 2020, unequal gender politics translate to women in relationships with men carrying out the lion's share of the emotional and practical burden of the household tasks. It may feel unconnected to sex, but it most definitely is not and can impact on our time for sex, our ability to prioritize sex, our feelings about our partner, the relationship, or our feelings about ourselves, as it did for Sandra. As we will learn as we move through the next few chapters, committing to more equity in this regard can be one way that partners can create the foundations women might need in order to cultivate and maintain desire.

The good news about all of this is that the effects of having young children don't affect every couple negatively and won't last for ever. In my opinion, the most important thing is knowing that this kind of change in your sex life is very common. This is crucial, as it stops you worrying that it's a problem with you, your partner or your desire. Hopefully, what you've picked up from this book so far about desire not being a drive, and being responsive to context and needing to be triggered, explains the impact of kids on your sex life to a T. Saying that, it's worth doing what you can to keep sex as good as it can be for now, and putting some effort into making it a priority – as you are by reading this book – so that you don't find yourselves in a place where sex has gone so far off the agenda that it's hard to come back from in a few years' time. This does not have to take a great deal of time and investment, which you'll be pleased to hear if you are currently running on empty and juggling thirty things at once. It can be as simple as a few seconds throughout the day or week where you relate to each other as *sexual partners* rather than as housemates or co-parents. I call this 'sexual currency'.

Sexual currency

'Sexual currency' is the sex science terminology often used to refer to the use of sex as a bargaining tool, or the relative value of a person's sexuality. I use this term in another context, as a way to refer to the amount of sexual charge or interaction between us and a sexual partner outside of actual sexual experiences. The distinction between what constitutes a sexual experience and what can be better considered acts of sexual currency is an arbitrary one, so bear with me on this. After all, as we discussed in Part One, one of the problems we face with our sex lives is our definition of what constitutes enough or 'proper' sex – and heaven knows I don't want to add to that already narrowly defined concept. But, if you'll humour me for a second, should 'sex' be thought of as any sexual act involving a body part of yours or your partner's designed to bring pleasure to one or both of you, then sexual currency can be defined as any way of relating to a partner which has the undertones of sex to it, but does not necessarily include a sexual act. This could be a brief but suggestive touch as you pass your partner in the kitchen, a seconds-long but passionate kiss before heading off to work, or just spending time naked in bed together not having sex. The litmus test is: would you do it with your aunt? If not, and it doesn't involve a sexual act of some type, it's sexual currency.

Let me use the analogy of eating to illustrate the point (I'm fond of food analogies for sex, in case you hadn't noticed). If 'sex' is equivalent to holding food and biting, chewing or swallowing it, and feeling the sensation of food in your mouth, and the fullness of it in your belly, then sexual currency is thinking about food, talking about food with others, meal planning, looking at food, remembering food you've had, sharing stories about your favourite food, touching the food before you cook it and enjoying the process of cooking. Using this analogy, we start to see the importance food takes on in our lives, even when we're not eating. We can also see that even when we're not eating food, it has time devoted to it outside of eating which undoubtedly adds to the experience when we do actually eat. Thought about food, anticipation or communication about food, adds to our eating experience in terms of both building excitement to eat but also by ensuring we know what we want from our food (and potentially, so do others). But when you consider the relational aspect of sexual currency (i.e. it needs at least two people to happen), you start to see how having high levels of sexual currency becomes more than the way we as individuals relate to something, but a way that, as a couple, we relate to and define each other and our relationship. We become a more sexual couple whether we are having sex once a day or once a year.

In the early stages of a relationship, we typically have extremely high levels of sexual currency. We spend large amounts of time kissing, making intense eye contact, hand-holding, complimenting, touching, giving affirmations about our desire, flirting, being suggestive by looks, comments, texts and emails and being physically close. If you watch a couple in the early stages of their relationship, you can see the high levels of sexual currency running between them. Their interaction is sexually charged, even when they are not having sex. Their relationship is defined by a sexual connection. The more this couple continue to act this way towards one another, the more they feel sexual towards each other, as this is the nature of their relationship, what it's about, it's the way they relate. It's a virtuous circle which results in more desire and more sex.

As relationships become more established, we generally settle into other, more sustainable ways to co-exist, as well as new habits. It would be rude eight years into a relationship to spend the whole time at brunch with a group of friends kissing, gazing into each other's eyes or whispering erotically changed things to our partner, to the exclusion of all others. Plus, after the first flush of lust, the intensity of those early feelings subside to pave the way for less obsessive and maddening feelings, and thank heavens, as if we behaved the way we did in the beginning, we might lose sight of all else in our lives and not have any friends to go to brunch with anyhow.

I want to impress on you that it's the habits we fall into regarding how we relate to each other that are crucial, if we are to consider the sustainability of our sex lives over the long term. Continuing to relate to our partners as sexual beings, not just as housemates, friends, or co-parents, is a way of making our relationship a sexual one, even in the absence of acts of sex. Continuing to share moments like this together reminds us that we are sexual beings, and that we are being looked at in this way by the other. Having moments of connecting via sexual currency, on a typical day or dotted over the week, provides us with natural, frequent opportunities to transition into being more sexual together, should we want to, by providing us with a scaffolding to move from the basement level (washing up, talking about our day) to the first or second floor (more of a sexual zone) naturally and without awkwardness, as, after all, it's *what our relationship is about and the reason we are not just friends*. Considering sexual currency as part of our sex lives rightly situates the performance of our sexuality on a spectrum rather than an on/off switch.

For some couples, sexual currency is ever present and, though it may have declined since those first heady few months of their relationship, they still feel there is a sexual charge between them that they enjoy indulging and intentionally nurture. For these couples, no matter how often they have sex together, they feel connected sexually, and find the transition from putting the weekly shop away to kissing passionately against the fridge an easy one to make. These couples may find a period of time without having sex makes less difference to their sexual satisfaction, as they are still getting most or all of their motivations for sex met via sexual currency (for example, feeling desired, feeling close, feeling excitement).

For others, sexual currency has become increasingly absent since those first months and this absence makes it hard to see their partner (or relationship) as particularly sexual. Compliments, passionate kissing, and suggestive looks are so absent that, even if you wanted to do them, they can feel awkward, and even if they are intended simply to convey attraction, they can feel like a clumsy initiation of sex. There's a vicious circle here, as the less you relate to each other in this way, the less your relationship feels defined as a sexual one, and the less sexual it is. The less sexual it is, the harder it is to transition into being sexual together, even if you both want to. You'll see why this is important once you have read about models of desire in Chapter 7.

Sexual currency is about the culture of our relationship, and what's good about culture is that it is fluid and shifting, depending on how the people within it act. If you are reading this and realizing that you and your partner only ever passionately kiss as part of sex, and never at any other time, or some other aspect of relating to each other mainly as flatmates or co-parents rings true, then the important thing is that you can create a change in this culture easily by starting to do something differently. The other thing that I'd like to say here is that although I've talked about two types of couples here, one with high levels of sexual currency and one where it's virtually non-existent, there's plenty of variation in the space between these two, even for the same couple throughout the course of a typical month.

To reflect on this more, ask yourself the following questions:

- Do I see my partner as a sexual person, and do I feel they see me in this way?

- Do we find any sexual interactions a bit stilted and a stressful signal of more to come? Or do we enjoy fleeting moments of flirting or passion as just that?

- Do we feel comfortable sometimes sharing sexual thoughts, fantasies or memories?

- Can we be sexual without it having to lead to sex?

- Do we ever passionately kiss when it's not a precursor to sex?

- Would I feel able to send an explicit text to them if I wanted to?

- Could we watch a sex scene on TV and talk about what was hot about it?

- How would you feel in your sexual relationship if you had more sexual currency but the same amount of sex? How do you think your partner would feel?

- What impact do you feel it would have on the sex that you have if the two of you had higher levels of sexual currency between you?

- What small things would make a difference if you brought them back/invested in doing them more? (This does not have to be a complete overhaul of how you relate to each other, as this is drastic and also might not feel authentic.) What do you genuinely miss but, for whatever reason, very rarely do?

- How would it make you feel about yourself or your relationship if you did these things more?

Remember those motivations for sex we discussed earlier in this chapter? Revisit yours for a second. How many of them could be met by increased sexual currency rather than sex? How about your partner's?

In my experience of working with couples who want to improve their sex life, improving sexual currency often brings drastic changes in how people feel about their sex lives, even before we've gotten into talking about the acts of sex itself. I'm not sure I've ever worked on desire with a couple who haven't benefitted from making this kind of change.

In Chapter 7 you will see how helpful sexual currency can be when it comes to desire, and why. But, for now, if the above questions have got you thinking, perhaps it's time to invest in your sexual currency a bit more. We'll revisit the benefit of sexual currency for future-proofing your sex life in order to deal with some of life's unexpected challenges in Part Three.

In this chapter, we have focused on the very obvious fact that partnered sex usually happens with someone else and, for this reason, if we want sex to be as satisfying as it can be and if we want to nurture desire, it's important to pay attention to how the relationship is helping, hindering or stifling our sexual connection.

Often in magazines, or in advice columns, the state of the relationship is referenced in connection with crucial dynamics, such as conflict, contentment, communication and respect, and these are all very important and must be examined. But it's easy to muddle this with an assumption that, if the relationship is generally 'good', then sex and desire should work okay, and this isn't necessarily so. What I'd like you to take away from this chapter is that the relationship context and its influence on sex are wider than an absence of problems between you. I'd like you to take away that, to truly nurture desire within a relationship context, we must consider how facilitative or constraining our relationship culture allows our sexual expression to be, how intimacy or distance helps or hinders our desire and how our motivations for sex and the complex and intertwining meanings we make of sex separately and together might be responsible for creating sexual problems, or promoting sexual satisfaction.

Take-home messages from this chapter

➲ Talking about sex is difficult, but couples who talk about sex more have higher levels of sexual satisfaction than couples who don't

➲ Talking about sex helps us navigate the inevitable changes in our sexual preferences, overcome sexual problems and keep our sex life good over time

➲ A difference in desire for sex between you and your partner is normal and not in itself a problem

➲ Desire happens *between* people, not *within* one person's body

➲ Understanding our motivations for sex (and that of our partner) is crucial for understanding the function that sex serves in a relationship and for maintaining sexual satisfaction

➲ Having sex for avoidance reasons, such as preventing a row or conflict, can lower desire over time

➲ Relationship dynamics such as the concept of intimacy can help or hinder desire, depending on the couple

➲ Some couples would find an improvement in their sex life if they spent less time together and invested in their own interests and activities

➲ Some couples would benefit from spending more time together, to create more emotional intimacy, especially with self-expanding activities. Giving each other the scraps does not count.

➲ Sexual currency can buffer against 'having sex' being the most crucial part of our sexual relationship

➲ Increasing sexual currency in your relationship meets some of your motivations for sex, makes you feel like a sexual couple, and provides a transition to move seamlessly into more sexual time together should you wish it to, but often falls off the agenda after couples have been together for some time

➲ To have a great sex life, many couples will need to prioritize and make time for these aspects of their relationship, but often our belief that sex should happen easily and spontaneously gets in the way of us thinking of sex as a part of our life that we should take care of

Exercises
Reflection – Understanding your motivations for sex

1) Spend some time reflecting on the last year, the last five years, and perhaps what happened in previous relationships, if you can remember. Write a list of some of your reasons for having sex, or ones you think may have influenced you even if you can't remember, with the aim of understanding yourself and what needs sex meets for you. Revisit Axa, if you like, or think back to the last few times you had sex.

2) Make a note of whether these are mainly 'approach' (to get positive rewards) or 'avoidance' (to prevent something negative) motivations.

3) Discuss this with your partner and get them to work on their list too. Show them this chapter so that they can get an idea of the kinds of things it could be. Get them to think about when sex isn't happening and what is it they feel they are missing out on.

4) Once you've done your lists, set some time to discuss this together and take turns sharing your lists. The person listening's job is to:

ⓠ not judge

ⓠ ask open-ended questions about the reason, for example: 'tell me a bit more about that' or 'describe that to me – what does it feel like, or how do you feel about us when you get that?'

5) Make a commitment to not having sex to avoid a row or someone else's upset, instead try to find other ways to meet these needs instead of sex.

6) Try out what it's like to focus on approach motivations, by thinking about positive things that you, your partner or your relationship might get from sex that could be nice, or perhaps write them down. Now that you are more aware of your motivations generally, try out what it's like to communicate what it is that you want when you want to be sexual and encourage your partner to do the same. In this way, you are both giving each other the opportunity to understand what the other might be needing, and having ideas about other ways to meet this if not sex. It's also possible that knowing why your partner wants to be sexual (for example, 'they want to feel close to me', rather than 'they just want to come') might make a difference to how open you feel to exploring your own desire.

Trying it out – sexual currency overload

This is an experiment for 'going to town', as it were, on increasing your sexual currency, to see what difference it makes to your sexual satisfaction, your feelings about yourselves as a sexual couple, your motivations for sex and sexual desire.

For this exercise to be most effective, you need to make a commitment to each other that the efforts you make to increase sexual currency won't lead to any type of sex together (in terms of sexual acts). Taking sex off the agenda allows you both to be free to take risks to create and be receptive to each other without expectation.

You will have an idea from this chapter what this could look like for your relationship, and it may be connected to things you did more of in your early days together. Do as much as you can of the things you know you both like but also throw in anything else you can think of to try. This might be reinstating passionate kissing or doing it more often, being flirtier, sending sex texts, complimenting each other's appearance, touching each other suggestively, flirting with other people, sharing sexual thoughts, fantasies or memories, touching each other in a more sexual way whilst watching TV or talking – anything you can think of.

Aim to 'try on' a more sexual 'couple identity' by doing as much of this as you can throughout the day. After a week or two, sit down together to discuss:

- ⮕ How easy or difficult was it? Did it get easier as you got more used to it?

- ⮕ How did it make you feel about yourself? Your relationship? Each other?

- ⮕ What impact did it have on your intimacy or closeness?

- ⮕ What impact did it have on your perception of yourselves as a sexual couple?

- ⮕ Did it make sex or desire feel closer or further away?

- ⮕ What else did you notice?

If it's been positive for you, make a commitment to build this into your sexual relationship from now on. Remember that life will get in the way from time to time and that this is normal. Ultimately, you have the power to change the culture in your sexual relationship.

6

Sex in our brains

The physical experience of sex might happen in our body, but our brains have the deciding vote in how we experience it. Our brains allow us to be in the moment, or can take us completely away from what's happening with a running commentary of distracting thoughts or judgements. These thoughts or judgements can take their toll on our pleasure and desire and, rather tragically, are often based on our learning, the absorption of societal messages, our experiences so far or the influence of the world around us rather than what might be *actually happening* in that moment.

In the last few decades, advances in sex science have taught us a revolutionary fact. Our physical experience of sex, such as how much sensation we can feel, or how much desire we experience, can be altered, for better or for worse, by our minds. This chapter will take you through how this might be playing out in your own sex life and how you can use this knowledge to your advantage.

First, we'll get a handle on what desire actually is as, without that, it's hard to understand how it can fluctuate and what our brains have to do with it. We'll then consider why your ability to pay attention to what's going on matters so much. Next, we'll cover how your brain is generating thoughts about sex and how these thoughts turn your desire up or down. Lastly, we'll consider the role of past experience in how we think about and approach sex and how crucial this is to future desire. My aim in this chapter is to move you to a place where you understand how your brain can be your best friend or your worst enemy when it comes to your sex life. Then, as always, I'll give you something you can do about it.

'Sex drive'

Before we understand how our brains help or hinder sex, we first need to understand more about the processes that influence our desire to be sexual in the first place.

Historically, sexologists and sex scientists conceptualized the way humans approached sex in a similar way to drives such as hunger or thirst. That is, as a universal human need that we are driven to seek out. The common colloquial use of the phrase 'sex drive' fits with this idea of something we just feel the need to do. We have all been socialized to understand sex in this way. But in the last few decades we have learned that the idea of desire being a 'drive' is not supported by science.[1]

One of the reasons for this is that, when something is essential to our survival, such as eating or drinking, and we go some time without it, we experience physical deprivation and so are driven towards it. Desire doesn't behave like this (something which any of you who are reading this who have not had or wanted sex for a while will be all too familiar with). In many ways, for humans, the longer they go without sex, the less feeling of 'drive' they have. This 'the less you have it the less you want it', model would not happen with any of our other essential human drives.

Human sexuality *does* have an instinctive component to it, as humans have an automatic response of arousal when we come into contact with things which our brains code as sexual (from now on I'll refer to these things as 'sexual stimuli'). This automatic response is pretty much outside of our conscious control and leads us to respond with some level of physiological arousal. Basically, there's a part of our sexual response which we share with other mammals, which is triggered easily by sexual cues, sometimes without our conscious awareness. Desire is kickstarted by this instinctive arousal, but has the potential to be sidelined or shut down completely by what our 'newer' brain – the parts of our brain which make us human – does with this information as it processes it.

The sexual stimulus could be the sight of a naked body, a sensation on our skin, or a sexual thought. Arousal is triggered, and fairly easily, in fact. However, our 'newer' cognitive (thinking) brain then uses complex processes, such as attention, learning and memory, to decide how much desire we feel. What's important to note is that the content of our learning and memory, and the kinds of things that distract our attention, are completely related to all the factors we've discussed in previous chapters. For example, if sex has been largely unpleasant so far, then our learning might be 'it's not worth it'. If our experience of sex is that it's more about someone else's pleasure than our own, we will not be that motivated to get involved. If we can't pay attention to sexual stimuli or our own physiological arousal because we are too distracted by other things in life, or all the things that could go wrong, desire won't follow. If we have a view that sex is largely lacking in reward or if our relationship dynamic is stifling of desire, our brains won't necessarily evaluate the stimulus of, say, a partner's kiss as erotic.

This is crucial to your new understanding about desire, as it's likely that, up until now, you've imagined that you should just feel like having sex instinctively (as a drive) and that, if you don't, there's a problem with you. What actually needs to happen for you to feel desire is something like this:[2]

HOW DESIRE WORKS

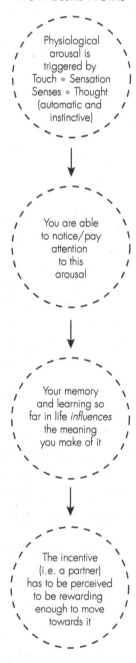

Physiological
arousal is
triggered by
Touch • Sensation
Senses • Thought
(automatic and
instinctive)

You are able
to notice/pay
attention
to this
arousal

Your memory
and learning so
far in life *influences*
the meaning
you make of it

The incentive
(i.e. a partner)
has to be perceived
to be rewarding
enough to move
towards it

So, your brain first has to notice this arousal (what's going on in your body or your mind), then make meaning of this, based on a lifetime of learning and experience (is this sexual? And, if so, is it positive and good for me, or not?). Before moving towards sexual behaviour, our brains will then do a quick calculation of the anticipated rewards of acting on our impulses or the anticipated costs (i.e. 'this will feel great' versus 'this will cut my sleep short by thirty minutes and mean I'm tired tomorrow'). A key factor and the final piece of the jigsaw is how much of a 'pull' the stimulus (a sexual partner) has. We'll come on to this later but, in basic terms, a new partner has more of a pull for us, as a rule, which is one of the reasons why people generally have more desire in a new relationship, as lack of novelty and predictability are disincentives to sexual motivation. A partner who we see as a 'sexual being' (as our interactions with them have high levels of sexual currency) will have more pull as a sexual stimulus than one who has started to feel like a brother/sister over time. Depending on how each of these aspects compete against the others, the outcome in terms of whether desire is felt or not will be different for all of us on different days and in different scenarios.

In this way, our brains act like a mental magnifying glass for desire. In one direction, they can amplify the strength of sexual thoughts, feelings and desire. But the flip side can just as easily minimize sexual thoughts, sensations and desire, through a process of distraction, negative evaluation and disincentive. This role that our brain has as a sort of data processor means that (even in any situation outside of sex) we are actually never experiencing true reality, just a filtered version of it based on our past experiences, social influences and unique thinking style. It is this filtered version of reality that can jeopardize our sex lives in a number of ways.

To help us really understand how all of this happens, let's look at the key brain processes, which are essential to our experience of desire, in more detail.

Arousal

We've covered the fact that the physical processes we associate with sexual arousal, such as changes to our body, particularly our genitals, are mostly automatic reflexes. This means that they happen to all of us without much conscious awareness when we come across something our brain has coded as 'sexual'. This process happens at a speed that indicates that it is bypassing parts of our brain that are more suggestive of conscious or cognitive awareness. When we come into contact with these *sexual stimuli*, which could be an image of something sexual, touch from a partner, a kiss, or the sound of people having sex, for example, our brains instinctively and automatically instigate an arousal response. You might not be noticing that this is happening in your body, but it is.

Much ground-breaking research by Dr Meredith Chivers and others has brought new understandings of the relationship between genital arousal and how this matches with what's going on in our minds ('subjective arousal'). This research has crucial relevance to desire, given that we now know that desire often emerges from arousal, not the other way around. For our desire to emerge, then, we must understand how our arousal works and what can put a spanner in the works of this chain of events.

Sex researchers like Chivers set out to understand just that – the mechanics of arousal. Over a series of important studies, participants in the study were wired up to machines that measure genital arousal. For women, this was done with a tampon-shaped probe which measured physical arousal by taking a reading of genital blood flow. The device for men is worn around the penis and does a very similar job. They found that when you do this in a laboratory environment and you show men and women porn, their bodies react physically with genital arousal, as measured by these devices. This response happens just as easily in the bodies of women who are feeling concerned about their desire as those who aren't. But how can the body and the brain be out of sync in this way?

In a 2010 paper, Chivers and her colleagues used the word 'concordance' to describe this phenomenon.[3] It basically means to what degree your brain and your genitals are in sync when it comes to arousal. What they found is that, when wired up to these devices, men's concordance is significantly higher than women's, on average, meaning that, when they are turned on in their bodies, they often report feeling 'turned on' in their heads at the same time. For women, this synchronicity between body and mind is typically much lower, on average, with great variation between women. Chivers and the rest of the research team put forward several theories to explain this phenomenon, varying from men's advantage in having a more visual feedback loop their whole life (hard penises are easier to see than engorged clitorises and vulvas), social restrictions on the acceptability of women's sexuality leading to women being less tuned in, and evolutionary strategies to protect women's bodies from harm.

Fascinatingly, more research from the labs of Chivers and others found that automatic genital response to sexual stimuli (essentially, what happens to your vaginal blood flow and lubrication when you are shown sexual images or porn) operates differently for women who identify as heterosexual than it does for people of all other sexual orientations. Men who are attracted to women, women who are attracted to women and men who are attracted to men all demonstrate the same pattern of their genitals automatically responding to a greater degree to their preferred sexual stimulus (i.e. gender). Not so with heterosexual women: their genitals respond to all types of stimulus, even if they don't report being turned on in their heads to it.[4] It's likely that this non-specificity has some relationship to concordance, as it suggests that (the majority of) women's bodies are not always matched up to what's going on in their heads. The truth is we don't yet know for sure why there is so much variation in women's concordance, but the evidence we do have suggests that being in tune with what's going on in our bodies is important when it comes to sex.

This makes sense, given our understanding of how desire works, in that it is first dependant on us being able to tune in to the arousal in our bodies. If we can't do this, we are unlikely to go on to experience desire. What the research evidence suggests is that the more what's going on in your body matches up to your feelings of being turned on in your head (i.e. concordance), the better your sexual response generally is.[5] Therefore, when your body and your mind are in tune it is good for your sex life. But what would cause us to not be in tune?

The role of attention in sex

A number of studies have demonstrated the devastating power of distraction on sexual arousal. Researchers in one study[6] wired men and women up to the devices which measure arousal, and showed one group porn and played the sound of the porn in one ear of the headphones they were wearing. In another group, they did the same, but in the other ear of the headphones verbal instructions were given, asking the participants to repeat out loud a sentence that they were hearing. In a final group, they were asked to do the same, but also repeat the sentence backwards after saying it forward once (a more complex task for the brain). What they found is that the more complex the distraction, the more it negatively affected sexual response. Listening to a meaningless sentence and repeating it or reversing it is certainly distracting, but as the researchers noted, in the real world, you'd never be distracted by repeating a sentence but rather by thoughts about your own life or sexual response. It's likely that these thoughts have more personal weight attached to them and so are probably more distracting still. Not being able to pay attention to what's going on is one of the key culprits for stopping us being in tune. The more out of the moment and in our heads we are, the less arousal (and therefore desire) we will feel. Remember your 'conditions for good sex' triangle from Chapter 3? This is where being in the moment is key for arousal, pleasure and desire.

This means that whatever is going on sexually, for example watching a sexual partner undress, a sudden intrusive sexual thought or the experience of a kiss, our physical sexual response is affected by how much attention we are able to pay to it. The kiss could be really hot, but if you are too busy thinking about the fact that you've got to be up in six hours, your body won't respond to it as if it is. Seeing a new partner's body for the first time might really do it for you, but if you suddenly feel fear when you see it, as you think 'what are they going to think of mine?', your attention is diverted from the sexual stimulus to these thoughts instead. Both the amount of attention you have for sex, plus the kinds of thoughts that divert your attention, matter to your arousal and, therefore, your desire.

This makes perfect sense if you think about it. Our brain has only got so much attention at any one time to devote to something, and as soon as something else competes for our attention it is divided. It's a bit like when you're at home streaming Netflix and someone else in the house goes online and your connection starts to buffer and stall, but *in your own head*. Generally, all non-sexual distraction is unhelpful: we want our attention to be focused on nothing but positive sexual thoughts and sensations.

Our brains are complex, especially when it comes to sex. Yes, they instinctively trigger the physical processes of genital arousal, and paying attention to this process is linked to how much pleasure we feel, but the parts of our brain that allow us to worry about sex and make judgements about it can reduce our attention to what's going on and switch off that arousal and desire by a process of anxiety and distraction.

Of course, all of us have streams of thoughts about anything and everything running through our mind at any point in time, as that is the nature of being human. It's also completely normal to have fleeting worries or moments of self-consciousness during sex (in fact, it would be odd if you didn't). But frequent thoughts like these that dominate our sex life can be enough to tip the scales, interrupting sexual response and negatively impacting on our sex lives over time.

What's also interesting about our thoughts is that many of the ones we have minute to minute don't stand out to us and we let them pass by almost unnoticed. Others we pay attention to, as they are stressful, exciting, worrying or in another way emotionally charged. It's the thoughts that can lead to more intense emotions, that distract us in the way those people in the porn headphones were earlier, by potentially leading to a further reduction in our sexual response.

Our brains generate thoughts like faulty time machines. One minute we're in the future, visualizing ourselves messing up that big presentation at work. A second later we're in the past, chastising ourselves for that time we said something stupid. Our minds can also do this during sex, worrying about what's to come and what it will be like, or remembering that time a person we were having sex with had a look on their face that must have meant they thought we were hopeless. We might allow ourselves to be in the present moment fleetingly, to notice that our partner is looking at us with sultry come-to-bed eyes, which acts as a sexual stimulus and immediately ramps up our arousal. But then we quickly get distracted by another thought – 'They want sex, but how could I possibly, when I've not had a bikini wax?' – and feel anxiety. We're not even just at the mercy of our worry about the future or the legacy of the past. Today's humans are also a product of intense social conditioning and comparison. The kind that convinces us that having pubic hair (which is normal, by the way) or seeing our skin wobble when we're in certain positions is such a crime that we'd be better off sacrificing our own pleasure to avoid it. The kind of social nonsense we talked about in Chapter 4, in essence.

Hopefully you can see by now that, as well as the importance of not being distracted, the thoughts that we have during sex themselves are important to our sexual response. In fact, research suggests that intentionally trying to reduce or amplify our arousal through our thoughts has an impact on our sexual response.[7] This means choosing to focus on thoughts such as 'they are really into this', 'I'm so attracted to this person' and 'this is so hot', which will turn up sexual response, in the same way that focusing on thoughts related to body image, performance or other negative aspects of sex will turn it down.

Let's talk a bit more about the kinds of thoughts we might have. They might be related to what the other person is thinking about us or what is happening. They could be self-critical thoughts about how we look or are behaving, i.e. 'they can see my cellulite' or 'they think I'm no good at this'. Our thoughts can be related to how close or far away we are from desire or pleasure, i.e. 'this is awkward' or 'I'm never going to come'. They could be thoughts about unwanted consequences from sex, such as pain, unintended pregnancies and STIs, or, alternatively, worries about not getting pregnant or sex being about potentially just going through the motions for people who are trying to conceive. We might also be plagued with thoughts about what we are doing and whether we feel it's acceptable or shameful, and whether sex generally is an okay thing to do. Lastly, we could be distracted by thoughts about the environment around us or worries about something non-sex-related, such as someone walking in or hearing, or tomorrow's meeting.

There's almost no limit to the types of thoughts our brains can generate during sex, one of all distract us or heighten our anxiety. Given our relationship with sex as a society tends to be shame, and tied up with anxieties about our performance or physical attributes, it's no surprise that many of us have the experience of thoughts about the things I've listed above impacting on our sex lives negatively. Negative thoughts during sex are also often related to many unhelpful ideas around sex found in society at large, rather than reflective of your reality in that moment. This is a real shame, right? You might predict that your partner is turned off by your stomach, as you've been sold an idea that only flat stomachs are sexy, and this means you start losing sexual sensation, when, in fact, your partner isn't thinking about your stomach at all.

Reflect on this for a minute. When you are sexual with someone else, what kind of thoughts swim around in your mind most often? It's really common for women to worry about things like how they look during sex, or to feel self-conscious when they are the sole recipient of pleasure, for example. Many women tell me that, when receiving oral sex, they are more focused on their partner's experience of giving them oral sex than being able to focus on their own experience of receiving it. The key thing about these thoughts (and I'm sure by now you've spotted this) is that we can trace many of them back to ideas about sex that dominate our society.

In my clinical work with couples and individuals, I notice that thoughts that cause problems during sex often fall into one of the following categories:

- How you look naked

- What they think of your genitals up close (particularly appearance, taste and smell)

- Their enjoyment and what they think of what's happening

- Your enjoyment – whether you're turned on enough or how close you are to orgasm

- Worry about experiencing pain, STIs, getting pregnant (or not getting pregnant)

- Self-judgement about enjoying sex itself, or the type of sex you're having or want

- What other people (family, friends, cultural or religious groups) would think

- Distractions from the environment (what if the kids hear/come in, TV on in the background)

⚫ Worries about other things (work, kids, lack of sleep, household jobs to do)

Once you've figured out which feature most for you (feel free to add other categories, if you have any), compare them to the cultural contexts and social messages influencing you that we talked about in Chapter 4. Research tells us that appearance-based distracting thoughts during sex, which reduce attention, arousal and then desire, are common for women, illustrating the role of society in our personal thoughts.[8] Our experience of being female is so tied up with Western concepts of being-thin-equals-beauty that it can be hard to switch off and let your body *feel* good rather than *look* good. Is this one of the main culprits for you? Is it because, as soon as someone goes near your genitals, you feel shame about how they look/taste/smell? Is it because you bear the majority of the household admin for the family and so feel the weight of all the jobs that need doing around the house and find it hard to switch off? Is it because you were brought up to feel that sex is shameful and you find it hard to let go and just enjoy it?

Working this out for yourself can be a great way to tackle these thoughts at their root, and to try to create a new reality that is based on how you really want to feel about these things instead. For example, given we know the impact that societal messages can have on all of our ideas about sex, imagine the difference it would make to how positive you felt about being a sexual person with sexual needs if you started to engage in movements which were all about women from all walks of life embracing their sexuality unashamedly. If you feel underconfident about your genitals, imagine the difference it would make if you followed social media accounts which celebrate vulvas in all their diversity. If you are too distracted by thoughts about the present that needs buying for the birthday party your youngest is going to this weekend to be present during sex, imagine what it would be like if this didn't feel like it was solely your responsibility and your partner held these things in mind in equal amounts. If you're interested in tracking these thoughts a bit more, so you can do something about them to reduce their impact on your sex life, there's an exercise which will enable you to explore this more at the end of this chapter.

By now you might be starting to get a picture of how complex our brains are when it comes to sex. Yes, our brains do instinctively trigger the physical processes of arousal, but the parts of our brain that allow us to worry about sex, make judgements about it, or not pay attention to it, can switch off that arousal or pleasure and get in the way of our sexual functioning.[9]

A word on psychological wellbeing and its impact on sex

We know that when people feel low or depressed, they tend to see the world through the equivalent of dark glasses, meaning that their view of the world, themselves and their future is negative. It shouldn't be surprising to hear that, as well as having negative thoughts about all areas of our life, if we are feeling very low we will also tend to have very negative thoughts about our own self-worth, attraction and sex lives. If we are feeling anxious, we might also experience anxiety in relation to our relationships and sexual lives. The physical manifestations that accompany anxiety or low mood can impact on our sexual response.

It's normal for all of us to feel low or anxious from time to time. But if you feel so low, or so anxious, that it's interfering with your daily life, you might benefit from understanding that this will impact on your sex life too, and working on your psychological wellbeing might also shift your experience of sex. Talk to your GP and let them know how you are feeling. You can be referred to an NHS psychologist or therapist to consider how the thoughts in your head are creating a picture of reality for you that isn't that positive and find ways to overcome this. It's important to know that there is good evidence that talking therapy can improve your mood, and help is available. It's also useful to know that some versions of medications used to treat mood difficulties, such as selective serotonin reuptake inhibitors (SSRIs), also have side effects of lowered sexual desire and difficulties with orgasm, so if you're taking one of these drugs and have concerns about your sex life, talk to whoever prescribed them and get their opinion. Don't stop taking them without discussing it, but if they are not helping the situation, it's worth knowing that there are other versions of these drugs that you can take instead.

Where do we want our thoughts to be?

By now, you might be wondering 'so which is it? A brain helping arousal and desire or a brain hindering it?' The truth is, it can be either, depending on whether our brain is focused on erotic thoughts and arousal or distracted by non-sexy or negative thoughts. The constant stream of thoughts we talked about related to all the learning in life we've done up until now will always be constantly circling through our heads, but it's the amount of attention we devote to those thoughts that will dictate their effects on sex.

Imagine your brain as a pie chart. You have a maximum of 100% of your attention to focus on the sexual situation in front of you. The breakdown of your attention might look something like this:

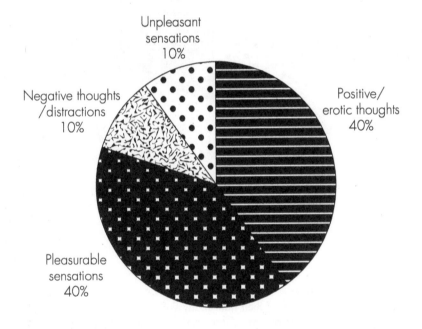

ATTENTION DURING SEX
HOW WE WANT THE BALANCE TO BE

Unpleasant sensations 10%

Negative thoughts /distractions 10%

Positive/ erotic thoughts 40%

Pleasurable sensations 40%

Positive/erotic thoughts – 'They look so sexy', 'I love it when they do that', 'They are really turned on by me'
Pleasurable sensations – touch feels good, vulva throbbing, feel of skin on skin, warmth
Negative thoughts or distractions – 'I can hear next door's cat – is it locked out?'
Unpleasant bodily sensations – feel cold, bit of cramp in left calf.

Versus this one:

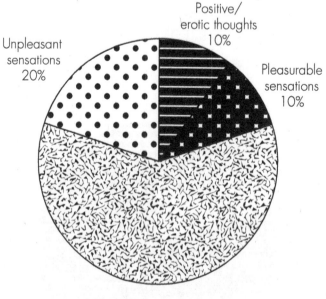

ATTENTION DURING SEX -
HOW IT CAN REDUCE OUR DESIRE

Positive/
erotic thoughts
10%

Unpleasant
sensations
20%

Pleasurable
sensations
10%

Negative thoughts/distractions
60%

Positive erotic thoughts – 'They are so hot'
Positive sensation – touch of their hair on my skin
Negative thoughts/distractions – 'They are too good for me', 'I look fat',
'My belly is wobbling', 'I hate it when they do that', 'I've got to be up soon',
'The neighbours will hear'
Unpleasant bodily sensations – some of the touch a bit painful, vaginal
dryness, lack of pleasurable sensation

Given that the amount of attention you are able to devote to sex is
important, imagine the impact of the differences in the two pie charts
above on the sex lives of these two women. But it's important to note
that both of these women might describe a completely different pie
chart on another day, in another situation, depending on their

'conditions for good sex' triangle and where they are with their psychological and physical wellbeing, mediated by their hormones and other physical states. These pie charts could also be the same woman days, weeks or years apart, or with a different partner.

For the second chart, if it's a pattern that is repeated over time, it's possible that the woman might get into a habit of the weight of the negative thoughts or distraction taking up more brain space than the erotic or her focus on sensation, making arousal less likely, sex less pleasurable, and having a knock-on effect on how much she wants sex over time. It's a bit of a Catch-22, I'm sure you can see. It can be worth considering this for yourself, just to get an idea of where you feel your brain is at for the most part, and whether there's a benefit in making some changes to how you use your attention during sex.

Before you start to worry too much about your wandering mind, it's important to know that being distracted by non-sexual thoughts is totally normal and happens to all of us frequently. In fact, in one study, 92% of people reported non-erotic thoughts during sex.[10] The key factor is the amount of time you spend distracted versus being in the moment. Exciting recent findings from sex science tell us that we can use our brains to change the size of each of these slices of pie and, in doing so, alter our sexual experience. I'll tell you more about this towards the end of this chapter.

Our brains have evolved to have such incredible capabilities, for example the ability to create art, music, and positive social move- ments that allow people to feel connected over an abstract common purpose. But our brains have also evolved to make links, associations and meanings in the events of our lives and to form judgements and future predictions for ourselves in ways that, at times, can make us our own worst enemies. This means that the nature of our thoughts and the meaning we make of them can turn down our sexual response like you can turn down the sound on the TV.

Understanding the role of learning

Our past learning has a huge part to play in our distraction, the content of our thoughts and, ultimately, our experience of pleasure, arousal and desire. But how does this process happen?

If you remember the summary of what desire is from early on in this chapter, it goes like this: we first need to be able to pay attention to what's going on and notice our emerging sexual arousal. Next, our brain decides what to make of it by drawing on past experience, memory and social learning. This helps us to decide whether to move towards this stimulus, or away from it. This motivation to move towards something, based on our past **learning**, the **reward** we feel it will bring to us and, crucially, the **attention** we are able to devote to it, is how desire works.

In Chapter 4 I introduced you to the role of social learning theory on how we learn and think about sex and ourselves in relation to it. In this chapter I'll be introducing you to more individual rather than social learning processes, and how these influence us when it comes to sex. Both are important for your desire.

The advent of early behavioural and cognitive theory in psychology were two key movements that provided us with some of this information. Behavioural theory came out of an era of science associated with testing cause and effect under controlled circumstances. Cognitive theory builds on this by explaining how our brains process information, build up memories, use language and pay attention, and how our behaviour is dependent on the interaction between these processes and the consequences of a behaviour.

In the study of this type of cause-and-effect learning, some theories evolved that are crucial to our understanding of how humans build relationships with the world around them.

'Classical conditioning' is the name given to a type of learning where we associate two things with each other. For example, after repeatedly witnessing its owner pick up its lead before taking it for a walk, a dog will learn to get excited as soon as it sees the lead, as it associates the lead with the feelings of enjoyment from the walk.

'Operant conditioning', meanwhile, is a type of learning where the reward for the behaviour makes a difference to our chances of wanting to repeat that behaviour in the future. For example, if the same dog gets a treat every time it stops and sits when approaching a road, it will be more likely to stop and sit at the road. When a behaviour is rewarded with something positive, we are more inclined to do it, and when it is not, we are less likely to do it (it's actually a bit more complex than this, but this aspect of it is all we need to know just now).

As these theories progressed, cognitive psychologists were adding to this mix by demonstrating the role of memory, learning, perception, language and attention to this behaviour–consequence picture. These key basic psychological theories are important when it comes to understanding our relationship with sex, given we are not instinctively programmed to seek sex, but rather our motivation for sex is under-pinned by noticing arousal and integrating this with our learning and evaluation of the situation.[11] Asking ourselves 'do I associate sex with pride or shame? Is sex emotionally and physically rewarding for me?' gives us some clues to this learning process in our lives thus far.

Pleasure (whether emotional, physical, or spiritual satisfaction) is a good example of a consequence that might make us more likely to be motivated to repeat a behaviour such as sex. Negative sexual experiences, such as pain, fear, embarrassment or shame, could add to the likelihood of us evaluating sex more negatively and being less inclined to do it (unless you get off on pain, or the experience of shame or fear, in which case it is, of course, a reward). Therefore, repeated experiences of sex which are either lacking in enjoyment or reward, or unpleasant, will reduce our desire for sex over time, by a simple process of conditioning. The orgasm gap is crucial here, as women simply have less reward for partnered sex than men when they have sex together. The value of the incentive (sex) reduces by negative associations or outcomes and increases with reward and positive associations.

Remember those motivations to be sexual that we talked about in the last chapter? These also come into the rewarding nature of sex (therefore strengthening our future desire) in terms of whether the experience of sex meets these initial motivations. For example, if you are someone who has an overall life goal of having a relationship characterized by intimacy and closeness, and you notice that you seek out sex when you are wanting to meet that need, the reward of an orgasm might be positive (and will certainly be useful), but the reward that might have most value is how close you felt during or after sex.

Another rewarding aspect of sex that can make a difference to our motivation and desire is how it impacts on our mood. If sex makes us feel better by relieving stress, offering distraction or making us feel valued, then this will act as a reward in itself. For some people, this is why sexual behaviour can start to feel out of control, as it is perhaps the only, or the most effective, way to make them feel good in the short term. If sex makes us feel bad, as we feel uncomfortable, bored, insecure, lacking in agency or as though it's about someone else, then this will act as a disincentive over time.

Other cornerstone psychological theories also give us clues about the involvement of our brains with our desire. For example, when the same incentive is presented in the same way over and over again, we develop a habituation to it, so it increasingly becomes less of an incentive. This is called 'opponent process effect',[12] and could well be one explanation for the finding from the Natsal team that people who have other types of sex without intercourse as part of their sexual lives report better sexual function, as the more different types of sex we have in our repertoire, the more variety we have at our disposal. It's also one of the reasons why our desire for the same person can lessen over time. These understandings provide us with the rationale for why we should be approaching sex, especially in a long-term monogamous relationship, as a buffet rather than the set menu of A then B then C, as, basically, the more often we eat the same meal in the same order, the less exciting and interesting the meal gets. After a period of time we might not be that interested in the food at all, as variety is associated not just with sexual satisfaction but also with the maintenance of desire.[13]

In contrast, the 'Coolidge Effect' is a psychological phenomenon describing how our sexual interest increases or resurfaces with novelty.[14] If you feed rats until they are full, they stop eating the same food until you present them with a different type of food, which they will eat even if they are full. Think of this as the equivalent of feeling desire for someone other than your partner. Understanding the role of novelty – and by this I'm not necessarily talking about nipple tassels (though also, why not?!) – but novelty in how you relate to each other, the roles you each play in sex, how you might use fantasy, and in the nuts and bolts of how sex happens, is crucial for the maintenance of desire.[15] Basically, our appetite for something predictable and familiar decreases over time, and re-emerges with something less predictable, known or expected.

Lastly, the interplay between behavioural theories detailing how we learn by association demonstrates how allowing sex to fall off our agenda as couples can make it harder to see our partner as a sexual being over time. The more we spend time with that person in a non-sexual way, the less we might see them as sexual. The tendency for our brains to make associations in this way is one explanation why couples who maintain sexual currency might see a benefit that couples who stop relating to each other in that way might not. This does not mean that it's harmful or dangerous not to have sex for a while, as you risk losing your sexual connection. Neither does it mean that you have to have lots of sex. But it does indicate that it might be *easier* to maintain a sexual association and see your partner as a sexual stimulus if you have ways of relating to each other that keep the association of that person as a 'sexual' being, whether you're having sex or not.

A word on the impact of sexual trauma

Sadly, many women have experienced non-consensual sexual acts, such as childhood sexual abuse or sexual assault, and these experiences can impact on mood and wellbeing as well as affecting our learning, memories, evaluations of sex and perceptions of ourselves as sexual. It's important to note that the effects of such experiences can show themselves in different ways for different women, so there is no one-size-fits-all relationship between these types of sexual experience and desire. For some women, this type of experience can dramatically affect their desire, through the activation of the 'fight or flight' response when triggered by sexual acts, words or memories or through a learned association that sex is harmful, deeply upsetting or about the abuse of power. For others, traumatic sexual experiences do not affect their desire in the same way. The key here is understanding which it might be for you and then acting accordingly with what you feel might help. If you are unsure what will help, you might want to consider asking your GP for a referral to a therapist who can help you to process the impact of the assault and help you find ways of managing triggers, limiting the sense of being out of control or fear when being sexual.

How can we get our brains working for us, not against us?

In the last decade there has been an explosion of research into the impact of learning to focus our attention during sex and the startling positive impact it can have on our sex lives. There is a growing and convincing body of research providing us with the solution for our wandering, self-critical minds, which have been sabotaging our sex lives. That research is in the application of mindfulness meditation practices to sex.

If you've not heard of mindfulness already, where have you been?! It's a technique that has its roots in Eastern spirituality and was brought to the West by a practitioner called Jon Kabat-Zinn.[16] Awareness of the usefulness of mindfulness in Western approaches to health and wellbeing has been growing since Jon Kabat-Zinn's successful application of mindfulness in the lives of people managing chronic pain, when medical treatments weren't helping.

Mindfulness is not a practice of *clearing the mind of all thoughts*, but one of *directing our attention in the way that we want*, and therefore not getting seduced into following emotionally distracting thoughts down a rabbit hole when they appear. In relation to sex, it's about paying attention to sexual sensations or the sexual thoughts that benefit us. In this way, the thoughts we don't want to focus on at that moment (the negative wedge of your pie) have less influence on our bodies.

In relation to sex, a growing number of studies have shown that mindfulness helps people be more in tune between body and mind and therefore improves sexual response. Several pivotal studies in the last decade have shown that women who practise mindfulness report an increase in their arousal, pleasure and desire.[17] In fact, research tells us that women who find it easier to have orgasms are typically more 'mindful' in everyday life, and find it easier to be in the moment in sex.[18]

I'm sure you can understand how this works by now. Mindfulness has been shown to increase our attention[19] to sex and move away from thoughts or distractions which are less helpful. It's a way of taking control of our brains and getting them to work for us, not against us. It fits perfectly into our understanding of how desire works and what can get in the way of it.

As well as helping us develop skills in focusing attention on sexual stimuli, mindfulness also helps us to notice our wandering mind and gently redirect our thoughts back to where we want them to be when this happens. It's a practical, in-the-moment way of shifting the percentage of attention in the pie chart we talked about earlier towards a bigger wedge of the positive. If we want better sex, sex where our bodies feel great, respond how we want them to, and with our mind staying totally in the moment, we now know that mindfulness is an incredibly effective tool to have at our disposal. We *can* have control over our wandering minds, no matter how self-critical our minds want to be.

This is precisely because desire depends on our ability to notice sexual arousal. Also, the nature of where we focus our attention. Our attention could be focused on predicting a negative outcome, i.e. 'they'll be upset if I don't come', or be totally absorbed in sensation – and I'm sure by now you understand what a difference it makes to sex which it is.

Dr Lori Brotto is one of the world's leading sex researchers looking into mindfulness, and she and others have demonstrated over several key studies in the last decade that, as well as being able to increase arousal and desire, mindfulness can also reduce sexual pain.[20] Mindfulness is a great way of becoming in tune with our bodies, and a great way of turning that magnifying glass of attention on to our sexual thoughts and feelings and away from distraction. It's beginning to become a cornerstone technique in sex therapy, and I have seen the power it can have to create sensations of arousal and desire in people who felt completely cut off from their sexual selves.

I'm hoping by now you can see what benefit getting your attention to work for you, not against you, during sex could have, regardless of how well sex is going for you just now. It's also worth noting, though, that all of us could probably benefit from being more mindful in everyday life, as well as in sex. It is clear that mindfulness works in many areas of health and wellbeing to a magnitude we're only just really starting to understand. The original studies were focused on pain management and showed startling results.[21] This is because, like sex, our experience of pain is mediated by how much attention we pay to it and the thoughts or attributions we give it. People started to take note of the impact that mindfulness could have, and so research began in other areas of mental and physical wellbeing. In the decades that followed, we gained solid evidence that mindfulness has a role in reducing anxiety and depression, managing impulse control in compulsive behaviours, improving how well children are able to learn or concentrate, and working against negative self-judgement, amongst many other things.

Throughout this chapter you might have recognized yourself as someone who is distracted or plagued by non-sexual or negative thoughts. Consider for a second, now you understand more about how desire works, the difference it would make if you could change this. The key thing here is that you can harness your brain to devote more focus to arousal and desire once you know more about what your brain is up to and how to focus it. Mindfulness is a skill that you can develop, and there is strong evidence that it will benefit your sex life. It's also extremely accessible, low cost and something which you can fit into daily life. What's not to like?

At the end of this chapter there are some tips in the exercise section on how to build your mindfulness skills outside of sex, then how to bring them gradually into your sex life as well, so that you can reap the rewards mentioned here. There's so much to say about mindfulness I would suggest that, if your interest has been sparked by this chapter and you'd like to learn more, you get yourself a copy of Dr Lori Brotto's recent book *Better Sex through Mindfulness: How Women can Cultivate Desire*.[22]

How the way we use language influences our thoughts

We talked about the importance of language and how it shapes our view of sex and how we understand the 'rules' of how we should be sexually in Chapter 4, but language is also important when it comes to how we (and our partners) talk about ourselves. It's important, as our choice of language is one of the ways we influence our thoughts about ourselves, our sex lives and what's possible.

We live in a society where we constantly refer to each other and aspects of ourselves with labels and categorization, which is probably based on our desire to categorize and group ourselves and others, based on social psychology processes. We label ourselves and others with fixed character traits that provide us with a shorthand to describe what we or each other can expect, but the words we use to describe ourselves and others can become stories about who we are that then define who we are, sometimes helping and sometimes hindering our journey in life. This generally means that the more we hear or repeat unhelpful stories about ourselves throughout our lives, the more imprisoned we can be by them.

How we talk about ourselves in relation to sex is important, especially as the backdrop to this is a medical and psychiatric system that has created language of 'dysfunctions' around sex, therefore giving us labels to use to describe what's wrong with us in the process. For example, the Natsal team found that a small minority of women in the UK feel they orgasm sooner than they would like. DSM has never had a category for early orgasm for women, even though this happens, probably as women's orgasm has never disrupted penis-in-vagina sex. But what would happen if we did have a dysfunction called 'early orgasm' for women? The likelihood is that more of us would worry about it, as then it's 'a thing'. What the medical world defines as a problem then provides the language for something to become a real-life problem, and it can be helpful to try not to get sucked into defining ourselves by such terms.

'I have low desire' is a good example of a label we might use for ourselves which can be quite limiting in the story of our sex lives, offering us little clue about helpful solutions, should we want them. It's used frequently in our culture and is the reason why those pioneering female scientists and sex researchers we talked about in

Chapter 1 argued against the old definitions of women's low desire, as they felt it was a useless label if it wasn't situated within the woman's social and relational context.

'I have a low sex drive' is equally as unhelpful. As well as implying that sex drive is a biological urge that is innate and fixed (which we have already established it isn't), it situates sex outside of mood, context or meaning, which takes away our ability to understand or change our experience of it.

A more helpful use of language might be 'I don't often feel like sex when I'm tired, stressed or when I know the type of sex I'm about to have won't be that pleasurable to me' or 'It's been challenging recently to have a type of sex which excites me.' Talking about desire in this way takes it out of who we are as a person (a 'person with low desire') and situates it in context, which not only makes us feel less of a problem but immediately provides a clue to a way forward. I mentioned in the previous chapter that I talk to couples about there being a *desire discrepancy*, rather than one person having low desire. The reason for this is not just because there is no norm to judge that person's low desire against, and desire should be thought of as a responsive motivation, not an urge, anyway, but because using this language positions the couple as equal participants in the challenge to overcome it.

It can be useful to pay attention to these labels, but also any others that we've adopted to describe who we are, as they can also inadvertently impact on our thoughts about sex. I work with so many women who have grown up with labels that hinder their sexual expression or experience of desire. Women who feel they are 'too uptight' as a person to ever really enjoy sex, too 'underconfident' to ask for what they want, or women who feel so defined by the label of having 'low desire' that they avoid relationships for fear of never being able to resolve it. For each of these women, the beliefs or understandings they then deduced about themselves as a result of this language resulted in behaviour which served as a self-fulfilling prophecy.

I'd like you to take a minute to consider any labels you or others use about you, your nature and your sexuality.

- What stories have you told yourself so many times that you believe them to be the truth?

- To what extent are these stories or labels connected to unhelpful social discourses about culture, race, age, gender, ability, size?

- How might stories, labels or language be impacting on your sexual life?

- Is it possible that these stories are either wholly untrue, or just more or less like you, depending on the circumstances you find yourself in?

- What possibilities does it open up for you in life generally and in sex if you reject these labels as facts about you that are set in stone?

My aim in this chapter is to give you an overview of how your brain, as the driving seat of your thoughts and other cognitive processes, might be impacting on your sex life at times, in a not so helpful way. We've understood the importance of our attention on processing sexual stimuli that might kickstart desire. We've also looked at the influence of our history and the world around us on the thoughts or associations we might have in relation to ourselves and sex. We've understood that sexual desire is how all these things come together to either motivate us to do it, or to have a cup of tea instead.

If there's one thing we can be sure of, it's that our brains are largely responsible for how sex goes and that, despite our brains being located within us, the factors which influence them come from outside of us. There's a reason this chapter follows the society and relationship chapter, as what we feel is expected from us, the dynamics of our relationships and the meanings we make of other people's behaviour become the fuel for our sexual thoughts.

In this chapter we've talked about the impact of attention and learning on the thoughts that we might have individually in the moment. We have the ability to improve our sex lives by becoming skilled at using our attention for us, not against us. We have the option to notice key themes in the types of thoughts that bother us most during sex and to try to find ways of ensuring they hold less influence over us. We also have the opportunity, now that we understand that sex is a motivation rather than a drive, to reflect on the benefits that novelty, a lack of predictability, positive reward and the opportunity to continue to see our partners as a sexual stimulus over time can bring to our future sex lives. We will build on this in the next chapter.

Take-home messages from this chapter

➲ Our brain is crucial to our experience of arousal, pleasure and desire

➲ Some aspects of our sexual response are automatic, such as physical arousal, but our body and our minds are not always in sync

- Negative or distracting thoughts can disrupt our sexual response by distracting us from the erotic
- Our ability to direct our attention towards or away from negative or distracting thoughts, and to pay attention to sexual sensations or stimuli, make a difference to what we feel in our bodies
- Sex for humans is not a drive but a complex interplay of our physiology, attention, learning and memory, leading to a motivation for sex
- Our brains generate thoughts all the time, but we can be distracted by ones which feel worrying and spend time focusing on them
- The more we tune in with our body, the more desire, arousal and pleasure we experience; and our attention can be harnessed through mindfulness
- Mindfulness is known to increase arousal, pleasure and desire and has been a key revolution in sex therapy over the last decade or so
- The language we use to describe ourselves can amplify the way we see ourselves in relation to sex, and stop us seeing how to create change

Exercise:
Reflection – What kinds of thoughts interfere with your enjoyment of sex?

Earlier on in this chapter we talked about how the things we think can influence our enjoyment of the sexual experience. We talked about the fact that there are often key categories of thoughts that come into our mind when we are being sexual, and that it can be useful to note which category your thoughts fall into most, and where these ideas come from.

In this exercise, pay attention to the thoughts you have during your next sexual experience with someone else. Afterwards, write down all the thoughts you had that you feel distracted you from your enjoyment, or were negative in some way. Once you have your thoughts written down in the same way they popped into your head (for example, 'They are looking at my stretch marks and will be turned off'), try to group the thoughts you have written into categories, as we did in this chapter.

You might do this over a few sexual experiences, if you feel you are someone who has a lot of negative thoughts during sex and you want to really understand this for yourself. Don't do this every time you have sex from now on, though, and please make sure that you also follow up this exercise with some of the mindfulness exercises afterwards. The reason for this is that, although understanding thoughts that are less helpful for you and questioning where they have come from and how you can challenge them can be helpful, as you have learned, it's not great for your sex life to get into the habit of paying attention to the less helpful thoughts during sex as a regular thing.

Once you have your categories, and perhaps find that it's one or two categories of thoughts particularly that affect you (for example, 'body image' or 'focusing on their enjoyment rather than my own'), spend some time writing a plan for how you can minimize the impact of this on your sex life, taking what you have learned from Chapter 4 into consideration. For example, you might wish to limit your exposure to airbrushed magazines and look at lots of social media accounts celebrating body diversity instead, or find other ways to increase your body confidence: attending a life drawing class which celebrates bodies in all their forms, say, or reading books about body positivity. You can change the script you are exposed to by lessening your exposure to the social messages that aren't helping and increasing your exposure to the ones that are.

Trying it out – mindfulness and sex

You will remember that mindfulness is a way of paying attention to something, non-judgementally, and being in the moment. It's also a practice of bringing our attention back to what's erotic, rather than to negative or distracting thoughts.

Mindfulness needs to be practised if you want to be able to develop the skills over time, and I encourage you not to rush this three-stage programme. The aim here is to first become skilled at mindfulness outside of a sexual situation, so that you become accustomed to directing your attention, noticing when your mind has wandered and bringing it back. When you feel confident with this, you can then start to incorporate these practices into your solo sexual experiences (masturbation), then into sexual situations with someone else.

Part 1: Download a mindfulness app and practise daily mindfulness outside of sex. The key here is to hone your skills in focusing your attention, being in the moment and gently and without judgement redirecting your attention when you notice it wandering. Given that mindfulness is a skill that needs to be practised, I'd be keen for you to feel confident at this level before you move on. It's up to you when you feel that you are confident to do so, but I would suggest you do this daily practice for a couple of weeks at least, if you are new to mindfulness.

Part 2: If you've been practising mindfulness a bit generally, by now you should feel more skilled in bringing your attention gently back to whatever it is you're focusing on. I now want you to move this on to two new mindfulness exercises, if you feel able:

- Choose to listen to mindfulness exercises that are centred on body scans and use your body focus to pay attention to genital sensation particularly (incidentally, you will notice most body scans you can download talk you through body parts then skip over the pelvis – fascinating from a sex-negative society point of view!).

- Bring this same technique of focus and curiosity in genital sensation to masturbation, as well as paying attention to sensations all over your body during self-touch.

Paying attention to sensation in your genitals/sexual sensations strengthens the mind/body connection and desire, and it's also great practice for focusing your attention where you want it to be during sex.

Part 3: After this, if you feel able, you can practise during sexual contact of any type with someone else. Use the same practice as when you're alone, but this time you can be mindful either to:

1) Your own sensations (i.e. what does your body feel like just now?)

2) One of your senses (pay attention to what you can touch/smell/taste/warmth/a visual image of a part of your partner's body)

As always, if you notice your mind wandering to a negative thought or a distraction, congratulate yourself for noticing it and direct your attention back to the present moment.

7

Gaps in our understanding of desire

I firmly believe that one of the biggest challenges to our sex lives is the gap in our understanding of desire. How can we expect to know how to enjoy our own sexuality and sexual relationships with others if we don't understand how our desire works? How can we organize our own sex lives if we don't have an idea of the relationship contexts that will fan the flames or put them out? How can we not feel that we are broken if we don't realize what's normal? This chapter is focused on redressing these misunderstandings by giving you the final pieces of the picture in order to complete your new understanding of desire.

Desire facts to blow your mind

You might remember that, in Chapter 2, we talked about the fact that, in research, many women report they feel little, or zero, spontaneous sexual desire (i.e. feeling like sex 'out of the blue') over the course of a typical month. These findings are important for several reasons. Firstly, we had previously been judging female desire by men's standards, and men typically report higher levels of this type of seemingly-out-of-the-blue desire. Judging women by men's standards and seeing men's standards as the baseline (hello, patriarchal bias!)

meant that women reporting not feeling any or much desire auto-matically looked problematic in comparison and were judged as such by the women themselves, their partners and their healthcare practitioners.

These new understandings, however, were so important because they told us that not feeling like sex out of the blue is normal for many women and therefore should not be thought of as a problem. The original question posed – 'How often do you feel like engaging in sexual activity?' – was measuring a type of desire we might call 'spontaneous' desire, which translates to *how often do you feel like sex with no obvious trigger for it?* Despite most women reporting 'rarely' or 'never', the majority of women reported that they still went on to experience arousal during sexual activity most of the time. What this means is that it is normal for women not to ever feel like sex out of the blue, and that this in itself does not indicate a problem with desire.[1] It also reaffirms our understanding that often desire follows arousal rather than being the trigger for it. This point is crucial to this chapter.

Given that sex scientists know this variability in how desire shows itself to be true and normal, why are so many women still concerned about their desire? The answer is simple. Women's arousal and desire work perfectly well for most in the right circumstances, but our current gaps in our understanding of desire stop us being able to create the right circumstances. Ironically, these gaps in our understanding even lead to us putting barriers up to those circum-stances when they do arrive, firmly closing the lid on the possibility of our desire emerging.

The history of sexology and our current understanding

So why do these outdated views of women's desire persist, leading women to feel that they are missing something that other women have in spades? In Chapter 1, I briefly introduced you to some key players in the field of psychology and sex research and how they contributed to our understanding of sexology, both in that era, and in the legacy of understanding that we've had since. You will probably remember Masters and Johnson – the pioneering researchers who observed couples in their lab having sex. Their observations led to the first time the 'sexual response cycle' was identified and presented as a uniform aspect of human sexual experience.[2] Though it was first developed by Masters and Johnson in the 60s, it was added to by Kaplan in the late 70s – the crucial addition being the inclusion of desire as the first stage, the precursor to all else.[3]

This is how it goes:

MASTERS & JOHNSON/KAPLAN'S
SEXUAL RESPONSE MODEL (1974)

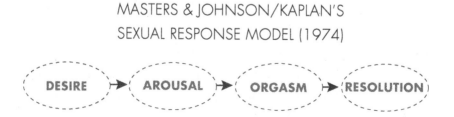

The model proposes that first we experience *desire*, a psychological urge to engage in sexual activity. This desire then prompts the physiological state of *arousal*, where chemical messengers are sent around the body by this altered brain state, preparing the body and genitals for sexual activity. The next stage in this model is *orgasm*, associated with the rhythmic contraction of the pelvic floor, uterus and rectal muscles, producing pleasurable sensations, then on to *resolution*, where the body returns to its unaroused state.

Now, this model has been heavily critiqued over the years for:

- The exclusion of anything social, relational and psychological, and therefore its assumption that sex is a simplistic biological process

- The assumption that people's experience of sex is linear and always follows this order (for example, orgasms always happen after arousal)

- That desire comes first (even though plenty of people describe having sex without desire and we now know that often what comes first is arousal)

- That it has been designed and based largely on male physiology and privileges male biology and experience over women's

You can see one aspect of this male-centric argument if we talk about orgasm. If this model were based on female arousal, it could go from arousal to orgasm back to arousal then orgasm continuously, given that many women are multi-orgasmic. We spoke about gender politics and their enormous influence on our sex lives in Chapter 1, but here's another example of it in action in sex science – for decades, women's sexual experience has been conveniently sidelined for a model that, essentially, fits men better. When Masters and Johnson observed couples in their lab, they observed this sequence in men, and also observed and documented variations of this response in women, but in their proposal of a final model they settled on one which was more aligned with male experience.

In my clinical experience, many men subscribe to the above model and say it fits quite well for them. If you have a male partner, perhaps show it to them and ask them what they think about it. It's a great way to understand their experience (and a good way a good way to start a conversation about how your experiences may differ). Research has found that a good proportion of men (and also some women) feel it fits for them too. There is nothing wrong with a person subscribing to this model.[4]

So, Masters and Johnson's and Kaplan's model first told us what was considered at that time to be normal. We feel desire – we act on it – our body gets turned on – we come – the end. As we reflected in Chapter 4, language that starts off in science becomes collective social and cultural understanding. It becomes 'truth' and informs our reality without us even realizing. Our conceptualizations of desire are the perfect example of this. The only model we had for decades told us *desire comes first*, that desire is present spontaneously, before anything else. The absence of this kind of desire then became one of the criteria in making a diagnosis of a problem with desire based on this model. What science and medicine dictate is normal filters down and becomes cultural and popular understanding. So that's what we take as our truth, that's what informs our sexual scripts, and that's what we then feel we fail at, if this is not our experience. It's the reason women incorrectly feel they have 'low desire' if they don't feel like sex out of the blue.

Despite a general trend for spontaneous desire to show itself in situations with new partners or after some time apart, there are some theories of why some women might experience higher levels of spontaneous desire in long-term relationships than others.

New, important theories of sexual response, such as the Dual Control model, suggest that sexual response is influenced by the interaction between two internal systems – 'sexual excitation' and 'sexual inhibition' – and that depending on the balance of these, people have the propensity to be more or less likely to engage in sex.[5] We can roughly think of this as what makes the difference between two people in terms of their 'arousability'. 'Arousability' in this context means that you might think about sex often, or feel more inclined to invest in or notice sexual stimuli and desire. These separate but connected systems are underpinned by both neurophysiological and psychological processes – that is, the roles of our body, hormones and brain and the role of all of our past learning and experience. 'Sexual excitation' might be described as how easy it is for a person to become aroused in response to things like sexual thoughts, images, interactions with others and bodily sensations. 'Sexual inhibition' refers to the tendency to lose arousal in response to perceived threats, such as reactions from others, distractions, negative feelings about sex, risk of unintended pregnancy or pain, or perceptions of transgressing social norms and values. Sex educator and researcher Emily Nagoski has made the useful analogy of 'sexual excitation' being akin to a car accelerator and 'sexual inhibition' being the brakes as a way of conceptualizing these two systems.[6] One of the aspects of sexual inhibition which has been shown to be particularly important for women with concerns about sex is something called 'arousal contingency',[7] meaning how easily you find yourself getting distracted from sex, or needing the conditions to be 'just right' to get and stay turned on. The more this is the case, the more it will interrupt sexual responses such as desire. Another aspect of sexual inhibition is being overly attentive to your own sexual function by focusing on worries that you won't get turned on or orgasm. For women, high levels of sexual inhibition are more predictive of concerns with desire, regardless of levels of sexual excitation.

I'm sure you can make some educated guesses from what you've read so far as to which types of experiences, learning and attitudes might influence your sexual excitation or inhibition in a unique way. The Dual Control model tells us that it's the interaction between the two that will make a difference to whether desire/sexual response flourishes or is extinguished, based on all of the other factors we have discussed so far as well as the result of neurochemical processes. Again, it comes back to the idea that desire is not a drive but a result of the processing of our learning, memory and attention, a projection of future consequences and rewards and how all of this interacts with our biology. This means that it's possible that if you're someone with high sexual excitation and low sexual inhibition, this might lead you to notice more spontaneous desire than someone with the opposite combination.

So, is your desire responsive or spontaneous? The truth is, for the purpose of this book and your sex life, it probably doesn't matter which it is. What you can expect is that, if you are in a newer relationship, having sex with (or fantasizing about) someone other than your regular partner, or have had a period of time away from your partner, you might have the experience of feeling like sex out of the blue. But there will also be some of you who *regularly* feel like sex seemingly out of the blue.

There will also be many of you who never feel like sex out of the blue at all (or rarely) and whose desire only ever seems to come from non-sexual motivations (wanting to feel close or other 'approach' reasons, such as because a partner wanted to) or as a consequence of allowing yourself to feel physical arousal first. For some of you, it will be a mixture of the two. What is key is that the context that you exist within (society, culture, your relationship and the messages you receive in relation to gender) will be influencing it.

There's a bit of a caveat here, in that current thinking in sex science is that there is no such thing as 'spontaneous' or 'responsive' desire and that it's more likely that all desire is *technically* responsive but that we may not always be consciously aware of the triggers for our spontaneous desire. What's important at this stage is understanding that both experiences are valid and normal, and there are plenty of factors in your life, relationships, contexts, circumstances and psychology which will impact on your own experience of it.

A new understanding

In 2000, a Canadian doctor with a special interest in sexual medicine, Dr Rosemary Basson, proposed a new model of sexual response for women, which set the path of understanding and research into women's desire on a new trajectory.[8] Basson's circular model of sexual response included many aspects that had been picked up by recent research, among them the importance of context, that the initial motivation for sex might not be sexual, the impact of the relationship and the importance of pleasure as reward. Basson's model also included the fact that many women in established relationships feel little 'spontaneous' desire, so they must be assumed to be starting from a place other than this. Basson questioned how fitting other existing models could really be if they did not include these aspects. She also questioned whether a lack of understanding about female desire was largely responsible for the high rates of women reporting concerns about desire in global studies.

The key points of the circular model are that women in established relationships usually start from a state of *sexual neutrality* (that is, without desire). However, the model suggests that if women are willing to seek out or be receptive to sexual stimuli, and if there are no negative psychological or biological barriers, they may find themselves experiencing sexual arousal. In this model, *only then* do they go on to experience sexual desire.

BASSON'S MODEL (2000)

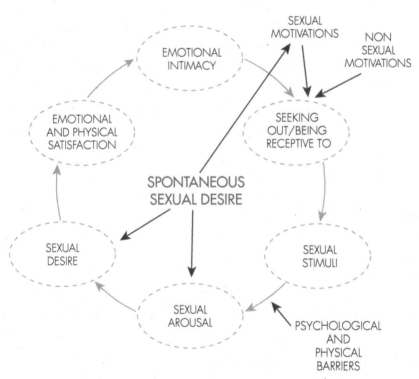

This means that we first must be receptive to the idea of desire (this is not the same as having desire), then have something to trigger it, and then there to be nothing that gets in the way of it. After this, arousal (physical changes) come before desire. Remember how this process happens from the last chapter? If, after desire, the sexual encounter is experienced as *physically or emotionally rewarding* (pleasure, orgasms, satisfaction), women report increased emotional intimacy directed towards their partner, and this makes them more likely to be receptive to or to seek out sexual stimuli in the future. Equally, a decrease in pleasure, satisfaction or emotional intimacy could negatively influence the picture and leave us feeling less receptive to sex (the effect of low reward).

This circular model, as you can see, makes provision for the spontaneous desire of some women, or some women in some contexts, at several points. It's important to remember that it's not the case that women in long-term relationships can't or don't experience spontaneous sexual desire in its own right. Some women report high levels of spontaneous sexual desire, just as some men don't. And some women experience spontaneous sexual desire from time to time, say once a month, which (for women not on hormonal contraception) can be linked to the period around ovulation and just before their period.[9] But it's not the case for all, and it's certainly not the three-times-a-week spontaneous desire that everybody feels they *should* be feeling, as described in Chapter 4.

Basson's model normalized the experience of non-sexual motivations for seeking out or being receptive to sexual stimuli (think of the list you came up with for your own motivations in Chapter 6). It may be these reasons, not feeling desire, which prompt a woman to seek out or be receptive to sexual stimuli. Following this, and as long as there are no barriers to this, arousal and desire follow.

The key messages in Basson's model are:

⊗ Women's desire is often experienced as *responsive* and can be triggered by being receptive to sexual stimuli

- Many things come before desire; desire is not first. In fact, women waiting for desire to come first might be waiting a really long time

- There are many different motivations for sex other than desire and, once women have decided to invest in sex, arousal and desire often follow

In my clinic, many women tell me that this model really fits their experience, and plenty of men do too. Does it fit for you? How might having different experiences of desire than your partner have impacted on your sexual relationship so far? Basson's model is exceptionally useful in helping some people understand how desire features in their life and where they can make changes that will make a difference to desire. For this reason, I want to focus on each part of the model in a little more detail, so you can really understand how it might fit with your experience.

Being receptive

The *seeking out or being receptive to* aspect has sometimes been called 'willingness', a kind of 'start-and-see-how-you-go kind of thing' – the problem, though, is when we're waiting for sexual desire before we engage in any type of sexual activity (and we often do this, as we have been led to believe that this is how things should be), we sometimes do the opposite of being receptive, by putting a virtual stop light to any situation where sex might be expected. We can even become hypervigilant to any subtle cue or initiation from a partner that they might want things to go this way. This stage can, therefore, be the first place our desire is extinguished, even before it's had a chance to catch alight, as in the case of Tori below.

> Tori knows that Dan always wants to have sex on a Saturday morning, as it's the first day of the week that both of them don't have to jump out of bed when the alarm goes off. She wakes up before him and jumps out of bed for a shower to avoid any awkwardness.

In the above example, Tori is hypervigilant to Dan's desire, is not feeling receptive and, as such, makes decisions to actively avoid any sexual stimuli. This can be a common experience when differences in desire have become a source of conflict. In contrast, in the example below, Meena is more receptive to sexual stimuli and this pays off in the gradual building of arousal.

> Meena knows that Roxy has sex on her mind when Roxy starts stroking the small of her back with her fingers while they watch TV. Meena doesn't, at that moment, feel like she wants sex, but she is enjoying the touch and is happy to let Roxy keep touching her in this way, as it feels nice. After a while, Meena starts to feel the familiar sensation that her arousal is building and, before she knows it, they are kissing passionately. At some point Meena starts to feel that she would like things to go further.

One of the biggest barriers, in my clinical experience, to being receptive to sexual stimuli in order to allow desire to emerge is the pressure that comes from sexual scripts – ideas such as 'don't lead people (especially men) on', 'it's impolite to start then stop', and that sex must unfold in a certain way (ending with a penis in a vagina). These scripts stop us at the first hurdle, as how can you enjoy a passionate kiss for a kiss's sake if you feel it will lead to turning a partner on, giving them the idea that you want sex when you (currently) don't

Dr Karen Gurney

and then, ultimately, when you turn them down? The truth is you can't, and in the playing out of these scripts opportunities for sexual stimuli (the passionate kiss), which might trigger arousal, are lost.

In my experience, women and their partners have to really understand the importance of being able to be truly receptive to experiencing desire by having a culture of high receptivity and low pressure when it comes to how they relate to each other sexually. In reality, the opposite often happens when there is a desire discrepancy, with one partner hypervigilant to being disappointed and the other hypervigilant to disappointing. Add this to the experience of less sex in the relationship than (at least) one person might like, and every kiss, touch or moment of being naked together can feel that it is loaded with pressure for it to lead to sex. For the person who has been feeling less desire, it can feel easier to avoid this rather than feel immense pressure for more. For the person who has been feeling more desire, the rarer these moments are, the more important it can feel for them to be responded to or to go somewhere. Before you know it, you're in a spiral of pressure and disappointment around something as simple as a kiss.

This is where sexual currency comes in, as well as the importance of how women have been socialized sexually to prioritize someone else's pleasure and not disappoint people. If you remember from Chapter 5, sexual currency is a way of describing the amount of relating to each other as sexual partners you do, the sexual culture of your relationship. Increasing sexual currency promotes a culture of enabling receptivity, by virtue of the fact that sexual stimuli are frequent and not in themselves signals of sex. Importantly, to be receptive to situations which might trigger desire, women need to feel able to prioritize their own sexual needs above someone else's, not fear 'letting someone down', and have the sexual agency to feel able to draw the line anywhere they like in the encounter without fear of repercussion.

Sexual stimuli

In the example of Roxy and Meena earlier, the frequency of this type of sexual currency between them acts as a sexual stimulus and will have an impact on how often Meena feels desire. Meena won't always feel desire when Roxy touches her back and kisses her in this way – for example, if she's had a stressful day and is preoccupied, if they've just had a row and she's feeling resentful, or if she's feeling tired. However, the more they have these kinds of interactions, the more chance there is that some of the time desire will be triggered. You might remember that sexual stimuli are anything that can trigger our arousal, whether we mean it to or not. Intentionally thinking about sex or fantasizing is a sexual stimulus, as might be a partner's attempt at initiation using indirect means. We might interpret something that someone (a partner or someone else) does as a sexual stimulus even if they didn't intend it to be. We also can't always adequately guess what kind of sexual stimuli might turn us, or our partners, on and they will be different for all of us, at different times, in different relationships. Also, sometimes sexual stimuli might be erotic for us on one occasion but completely turn us off the next. Remember Tori from just a second ago? Let's imagine that Tori was feeling receptive and didn't jump out of bed on Saturday morning.

Tori interpreted Dan's behaviour in bed on a Saturday morning as a sexual stimulus, as he often rolled over to her half asleep, ran his hands over her naked stomach and kissed her neck. She enjoyed the sensation of his hands on her body, and there was something

> about him doing this in bed when they were sleepy and warm
> that she found really sexy. Tori had woken up ten minutes earlier
> than Dan, and in this time had wondered whether they might
> have sex, given it was Saturday and they had nowhere to be. In
> these ten minutes before Dan awoke, Tori indulged in sexual
> thoughts and found herself feeling arousal and some desire before
> he'd even woken up.

In this example, Tori has the sexual stimuli of being physically close to Dan and the experience of enjoyable touch from him, as well as her own inner world of sexual thoughts, which has acted as a kickstarter for her desire. In the first example, Tori rarely got to experience these sexual stimuli as she had already got out of bed in anticipation, knowing it was coming and second-guessing where Dan wanted it to go – somewhere she didn't, at that moment. In the second example, Tori was feeling receptive and had the opportunity for arousal and desire to be triggered.

What about Dan? There are several things that could have been going on for Dan. Firstly, he may not have intended this touch and kiss to be any more than that; it might just be his way of connecting and enjoying Tori's body for five minutes before they get out of bed. It's also possible for Dan that this touch might be a way he stimulates his own arousal and desire, if he also wanted to feel like sex (remember, men are not from Mars). Finally (and even in combination with the last reason), it's possible that Dan could have been communicating with Tori, via indirect sexual initiation, that he would like them to be sexual together. Remember also that Dan would have had his own reasons or motivations to be sexual, and it is likely that Tori's reaction of seeming to want to avoid him and jump out of bed or, alternatively, enjoying five minutes of touch or a kiss, might have made an enormous difference to his needs being met, depending on the reasons he was prompted to connect with Tori in that way.

In Chapter 5, we considered the role of a particular communication called 'sexual initiation' and that it could be direct or indirect. Alongside 'accidental' sexual stimuli (for example, seeing a sex scene on TV that you find hot) and increasing sexual currency (an intentional way of relating sexually, such as reinstating passionate kissing, which at times will act as such), 'sexual initiation' is a direct attempt at using sexual stimuli to communicate something to someone else.

Let's use Amy and Mark as example here to help us. Look at this list of how sexual initiation features as a sexual stimulus in their relationship. At the bottom of the list we can see the sexual initiations that don't act as adequate sexual stimuli for Amy. In fact, she finds them a turn-off. In the middle are the sexual stimuli that sometimes Amy might be receptive to, that sometimes work for her and sometimes don't, depending on what else is going on. The few at the top represent the things which Amy has never shared with Mark which she thinks, if she was feeling receptive, would really work for her as sexual stimuli.

- Mark sending her explicit texts or images about what he would like to do to her that evening

- Mark making the effort to buy himself new underwear and surprising her by wearing it

- Mark offering to give her a whole-body massage but insisting it mustn't lead anywhere

- Mark looking all hot, sweaty and sporty when he comes in from a run

- Mark running his fingers through her hair absent-mindedly while they are watching TV

- Watching Mark at a party flirting a bit and being confident and fun

- Mark saying, 'It's been a while – how about tonight, then?'

- Mark coming up behind Amy and grabbing her breasts roughly while she is getting ready for work

We might want to nurture our responsive desire and be receptive to sexual stimuli so that we can go on to experience sexual arousal and desire, but as well as considering our exposure (and our ability to notice or pay attention) to sexual stimuli on a broader level, it is also worth considering:

- Have we got stuck in a non-sexy rut around sexual initiation?

- Does our relationship actually feature very little sexual stimuli these days?

- Might we even feel unskilled at knowing how and what to do to take things further, even if we want to?

- Is one of us holding up a virtual stop sign to these triggers even before they've started?

- Are there things that we don't know about each other that might work very effectively as sexual stimuli and sexual initiation if we were able to discuss them?

✪ What are the things we wish we could say to each other about what we'd really like the other to do / try?

Reflect on this for a second. Is there one thing your partner does when you think they'd like sex that doesn't work for you or really closes you down psychologically for more sexual intimacy? Are there things you would love them to do that you think would work for you but you've never asked for? How do you indicate a want for sexual intimacy with your partner (verbally? non-verbally?) and how do you think they feel about this?

'My ex used to kiss me in a certain way, but it got "samey" and, in the end, I hated it. He wouldn't do anything else and sex really dried up for us as I found the predictability a real turn-off.' (Amanda)

'My partner simply says, "Fancy a shag?" It makes me feel annoyed rather than anything else. I never really know how to let him know when I do feel like sex – I'm at a total loss. I just kind of hope he picks it up.' (Serena)

'I don't think my partner has any idea there are things that really turn me on when they do them, and things that really don't.' (Roberta)

One of the exercises for you to choose from at the end of this chapter will be to consider this for yourself and discuss it with your partner. It's a really important aspect of the model, as if you are feeling receptive but the things that either one of you are currently doing or saying is stopping your arousal and desire from emerging, it's crucial to address it.

It's also vital that we don't see ourselves or our partners as having failed or got something wrong here. The fact is, it's both people's responsibility to find a way to communicate about what works when it comes to sex, and if we're not doing that effectively, we can't expect to mind-read what each of us might like. Remember that we have also reflected that sex can be hard to talk about, so it's no wonder we can be out of sync with these things sometimes, especially given our wants and preferences can change over time. Sarah and Clio, below, are examples of how actions intended to be sexual stimuli by one partner can actually become turn-offs over time, or barriers to desire, if not addressed.

Sarah was in a relationship with Oli. When Oli was feeling like sex, he would come up behind Sarah and put his hands between her legs over her clothes. He'd learned to do this in a previous relationship, when an ex-partner had often responded positively to it. Sarah found it too much and really offputting, but had never told Oli for fear of hurting his feelings. Instead of acting as a sexual stimulus to her, this actively got in the way of Sarah's desire.

Clio was in a relationship with Abi. Clio and Abi had lots of physical affection but very little kissing or sexual contact in the months between when they were sexually active. One of the things Clio found hard is that it was clear to her when Abi wanted to initiate sex because she started talking in a different voice. Clio found this 'baby' voice quite infantile and unsexy but went along with it as she didn't want to upset Abi and knew that Abi was just trying to communicate something that was hard for both of them to talk about directly. They would often get through this initial awkwardness and both end up feeling connected sexually, but it never felt like the most comfortable start.

Sexual stimuli are not all about another person and what they do or don't do. We know that, for many women, fantasizing or thinking about sex acts as a sexual stimulus, as does watching porn, reading or listening to erotica or talking about sex with others. Some women report that there may be certain types of touch, smell, music or memories which act as triggers for them. Reflecting on and experimenting with discovering this for yourself can be useful information in regard to understanding your own desire. It can also be a revelation to see what happens to your arousal and desire if you expose yourself to a sexual stimulus, such as reading or listening to erotica or watching porn, as, in my experience, it helps women in two ways. Firstly, to understand that their responsive desire is working as it should and that, therefore, they are normal. Secondly, to understand that, if this is the case, there is something else going on with a partner that is getting in the way. This could be the notion of having not previously been receptive for the reasons we have mentioned. It could be connected to a lack of sexual stimuli due to having little time together or being out of the habit. It's also possible that this part of the model does go to plan, then something else kicks in to interrupt desire.

Psychological barriers

In the last chapter we looked in detail at how what is going on in our minds affects what's happening in the moment with sex. You will remember that there are several key psychological barriers, based on the attention we are able to pay to our arousal or our ability to be in the moment, the content of thoughts we have related to sex and how they add to this, and the learning or associations we have about sex related to every element of our sex and relationship history to date.

By now you should have a pretty good idea of the impact of what's going through your mind during sex. You'll also understand how negative thoughts about ourselves, sex and our bodies or not being able to pay attention to the good stuff turns down the intensity and even stops sexual arousal (and therefore prevents us from feeling desire). In the example of Andie, below, there were high levels of receptivity, sexual currency and therefore sexual stimuli, but there were psychological barriers that threatened to dampen her desire.

Andie often felt open to the idea of sex happening, and she and her partner created loads of opportunities for sexual stimuli in their relationship – they often kissed for the sake of kissing and frequently spent lots of time in bed together talking, laughing and with close physical contact. However, as soon as Andie had the thought that she or her partner might want it to go further, she was plagued with a whole host of worries about herself and her body. These were often focused on body image in one way or another. She worried that she didn't have the right underwear on, that it had been a while since she'd showered, how much body hair she had right now and what her body would look like in this light. Sometimes she'd notice that she'd almost have to battle through these thoughts until the point came where she noticed that she felt arousal and desire kick in. When this happened, she suddenly had the experience that these thoughts had faded into the background and desire had taken over.

A key psychological barrier we haven't covered in detail so far, which I want to draw your attention to at this stage, is expectation and pressure. There's nothing like feeling we have to do something or that something is expected of us to make that thing less enticing, and sex is no different. If we feel every kiss has to lead to sex, and if we feel that every time we have sex it has to lead to a certain type of sex, desire takes a hit. In my experience, expectation and pressure for a foregone conclusion are two of the key ingredients for a less than satisfactory sex life. The cultural phenomenon of 'blue balls' that we discussed in Chapter 4 is crucial here, as feeling as though 'we've started something so we have to finish it' (especially if this is privileging one person's needs over another) is just not great for long-term desire. Similarly, wedding nights, date nights, weekends away and nights in hotels can all have a similar effect.

The flip side of this is that anticipation can build desire and shouldn't be underestimated as a tool at your disposal to trigger it, and we talked about this when we covered scheduling physical intimacy. The key difference here is that pressure and predictability are about a foregone conclusion; anticipation is building excitement for something that may or may not transpire. Take a minute here to consider how pressure, predictability or anticipation feature in your sex life, alongside any other problematic thoughts or distractions you identified in the last chapter. The way to overcome this potential psychological barrier is to create a culture of low pressure between you and your partner. This means creating situations of physical or emotional intimacy which trigger desire but to have a solid agreement that this need not lead to a certain conclusion. I often explain to couples that I'd like them to move towards a 'trivial and often' idea of sexually relating, rather than 'rarely and crucial'. This, I find, can often require a complete shift in understanding for most couples, but once they are able to see the results that this low-pressure/ high-frequency way of sexually relating brings, it can often have a remarkable impact on their sex life moving forward.

Circumstantial barriers

In Chapter 2 I introduced you to the interesting fact that we are having less sex as a nation than we have ever had before. In my opinion, couples often don't give enough credit to the impact of their individual life circumstances on their sex life. It's so important to examine this, and it's one of the easiest things to change. Circumstantial barriers such as these are not named explicitly as part of Basson's model, but they would fit under the heading of psychological barriers, or as part of the wider context of the relationship. I encourage couples to think explicitly about the practical aspects of their life that dampen desire.

There's nothing more powerful and freeing than a couple who feel that their sex life is doomed due to some kind of incompatible desire problem realizing that they simply don't prioritize sex and that if they did, it might be different. The information this provides for a significant and meaningful change can be relationship-changing. They may not have come to this understanding before, as they believed that desire and sex should just happen spontaneously and 'naturally', without effort.

You might remember Alexandra and Will from Chapter 5, whose schedule for diet and exercise prevented them from having any time for their sexual relationship. Katy and Ryan, below, reached a similar conclusion.

Katy and Ryan had a realization that their schedules had no space for sex in them, and their expectation that sex should happen randomly and spontaneously when they didn't see each other alone that often was probably not that realistic. They made a decision to sacrifice one night a fortnight that was Katy's yoga

night and which Ryan usually spent with friends to really connect emotionally and physically, to create the right kind of
environment, space, time and conditions for sex. They didn't
always have sex on these nights, but more often than not they
did. Making space in their schedule meant other things had
to give, but it was a sacrifice they felt was worth making. This
solution was not apparent to them until they understood how
desire worked.

When there are practical factors, such as time, which get in the
way of desire emerging, the options are to choose to prioritize sex in
your life and to devote regular time to your relationship in a way that
works for you both (a compromise might also be required here)
or to accept that your sex life can't happen the way you'd like it to,
as life gets in the way, and rest safe in the knowledge that this
doesn't mean there is anything wrong with either of you, or that your
relationship is doomed.

Physical barriers

We discussed physical barriers in the form of prescribed medication
use, tiredness and hormonal changes in Chapters 5 and 6 when
we discussed the impact of having children, as well as low mood
and anxiety.

However, another physical factor which we haven't talked about so
much yet is the experience of painful sex. Penetrative sex can be
uncomfortable for all of us from time to time if we're not turned on
enough, if the position isn't great for us or if we don't use enough
lube for vaginal or anal penetration, and, as a rare occurrence, this is
nothing to worry about. However, around 7.5% of women in the UK

experience pain either from penetration, or from touch to the vulva, and this can drastically impact on sexual satisfaction and the desire to have sex.[10] The impact of pain is linked with the associations and learning we make, as discussed in the last chapter. If something isn't rewarding, we are less likely to do it, but if something leads to a negative consequence, such as pain, we are even less likely to do it than if it's just not rewarding. Sex should not hurt and, if this is something that you experience, go to your GP and let them know so that they can refer you for an investigation and so you can access support (typically, once medical causes for pain have been ruled out, this would be for sex therapy and pelvic-floor physiotherapy) to help you overcome it.

Arousal and desire

In the last chapter, we learned that having our brain and body in sync when it comes to arousal is called 'concordance' and that there is evidence that concordance is associated with better sexual function. One of the key aspects of the circular model is that arousal comes before desire. In fact, the process of noticing our own genital arousal and the other bodily changes and pleasurable sensations that come with it can often be what triggers our psychological desire.

This means that it is possible that women might not be noticing their own arousal, which might, for some, be a missed opportunity to kickstart desire. This concept is further evidenced by some of the research coming from the lab of Dr Lori Brotto and her colleagues, who, as you know, have found that women who pay attention to genital sensation using mindfulness have higher levels of concordance, arousal and desire after practising mindfulness regularly.

The other interesting aspect of genital arousal is that, when I work with women in therapy around their concerns about 'low sex drive' and I ask them whether they notice any genital tingling, throbbing and wetness over the course of a typical month, perhaps in response to something they've seen, read or thought about, they often say that, actually, they have. If they are not sure, sometimes I set them a task to do where I ask them to pay attention to this over the next few weeks, and they very rarely return saying they haven't noticed it. This often leads to a conversation about how they equate this with their perception of having little or no sex drive. These conversations can be very useful, as they often turn into a realization that the problem might not be about experiencing arousal or even desire but experiencing arousal and desire *directed at or in response to their partner, at convenient times of the day, or feeling confident or motivated to turn their own physical urges into the action of having sex with someone else.*

It's also interesting when women understand that their desire is often responsive to this arousal, to see whether they want to try and experiment with triggering it, to recognize and learn to trust this process in action. They could do this by watching porn, using fantasy or listening to or reading erotic stories, for example. It can be incredibly reassuring, as well as crucial for developing more of an understanding of your own desire, to realize that desire is triggered easily when the time is invested in doing so and the circumstances are favourable.

Practising this alone can also be a great way of understanding how your arousal and desire works, with sexual stimuli that work for you, and without any of the interfering psychological barriers. At the end of this chapter you'll find exercises to try out related to generating and amplifying arousal, so that you can learn more about this process, then make it work for you in a way that benefits your sex life.

In the circular model, the psychological state we might call responsive desire more often comes at this stage, after all these other things have happened. This means that waiting for desire to happen first as a way of running your sex life might not be all that useful for many women. It might also mean that, for many women, waiting for spontaneous desire might mean they are waiting a very long time.

Only when all the other circumstances are in place (erotic stimuli, an absence of psychological or physical barriers) should we really start to worry about our desire and arousal if they are not happening. I've only met a few women in my career who fell into this category, as opposed to several hundred who found no problems triggering desire once the other aspects were considered.

Emotional and physical satisfaction

Sex is not all about orgasms, and certainly Basson usefully frames 'emotional and physical satisfaction' as a broader definition of having enjoyed the experience. However, as you learned in the last chapter, having less pleasure during sex, or not enjoying it for other reasons, will limit the positive consequences and reduce desire over time. In Chapter 3 we talked about the orgasm gap between women and men when they have sex together. The orgasm gap is crucial to desire and, hopefully, when we looked at the importance of learning and memory for us to feel incentivized to be sexual, that explained why. Put simply, our desire flourishes, or is inhibited, by the amount of pleasure or satisfaction we experience.

Making sex mutually satisfying is not a goal that is out of reach for ANY couple, and couples who allow their sex lives to move towards something that benefits male biology and pleasure over women's should expect desire to decrease over time. This is more common than you'd think in relationships between women and men, for the reasons we have previously mentioned in how we view sex and gendered roles in relation to it. It is less common in relationships between women, and this is backed up by the data of the higher levels of sexual satisfaction for women in same-sex relationships.

If sex has become less frequent and less pleasurable, this will need to be addressed to avoid a potential decline in desire over time. Sex that doesn't always end in penetration can feel like a big culture shift for most heterosexual couples, especially if you've been having sex the same way for ages. This means that how we have sex, or what we see as sex is crucial for sexual satisfaction, especially for male/female couples. It takes a significant shift in understanding and, ultimately, a greater awareness to make a change away from something that has become routine for you. The risk, though, is that, without this shift, it's possible that your sex life might lose its charm over time due to habituation, predictability and lack of novelty reducing the rewards that sex has to offer.

Other rewarding aspects of sex outside of orgasms could include, for example, feeling attractive, finding it erotic, feeling connected, feeling close, having fun together or feeling free to express your sexuality. The more these things are happening, as you can see from the model, the more likely it is that the experience will be satisfying and reinforce future desire. Reflect on your 'conditions for good sex' from Chapter 3. It's the presence of these things that will make a difference here. But if these things aren't happening, if sex is lacking in reward generally, not just in orgasms, then this might need to be addressed.

Emotional intimacy

The circular model suggests that the positive consequence of sexual activity featuring emotional and physical satisfaction is increased emotional intimacy with a partner, leading to a sense of closeness and wellbeing. In contrast, it can be assumed that a lack of emotional and physical satisfaction from sexual activity might result in a lowered sense of sexual intimacy and connection over time.

This is important to the model, as the level of emotional intimacy feeds into the likelihood that the woman might feel receptive, or not, to future sexual stimuli. This allows women to be open to the idea of sex for non-sexual motivations, as with those mentioned in earlier chapters. However, a less rewarding version of this circular response might lead to a situation where sexual neutrality is more difficult, and it may become more challenging, therefore, to feel motivated to be sexual, or to feel receptive to sexual stimuli over time. Consider for a moment when you feel most emotionally intimate with your partner and what it is that facilitates this feeling. For some of you, it will be about time together to really connect, for others it will be about good communication and feeling listened to, for others it will be about having fun together. Maximizing these aspects of your relationship by making time to create opportunities for them, or simply treating them as important and essential to nourish, is key.

How does your desire work?

At this stage you can probably see that, over the course of your life, there may have been be a range of ways you've experienced desire (based on what we know about desire from sex science). The first is frequent thoughts of sex out of the blue, and although this is more common in the early stages of a relationship, and more common for men, some women certainly identify with this as a way their desire works. More likely, perhaps, might be a pattern of rarely noticing yourself thinking about sex or feeling like sex out of the blue, but if you read, watch or think about something erotic you noticing arousal in your body, which you may or may not act on. Or perhaps you very rarely think about sex but notice that, once you've let yourself be open to it and started some kind of sexual touch, kiss or act with a sexual partner, desire usually, or always, follows. For some people there may be a mixture of times when they feel like sex out of the blue, times when they are motivated to have sex for another reason and actively seek out sexual stimuli in the absence of feeling desire, and times when they are receptive to sexual stimuli and happy to see if desire builds. All of these manifestations of desire are normal.

Bringing this all together – Amy and Mark

Amy felt that she was someone with a low sex drive and she was often aware that she didn't meet the three-times-a-week feeling-like-sex thing she thought she should. She very rarely thought about having sex with Mark, but when she did, which was about every two months, she acted on it by showing him some kind of signal that she wanted to be sexual (like wearing nothing to bed) and he usually responded. When she did this, and they had satisfying sex, she often thought afterwards: 'That's was great – we should do that more.'

The rest of the time, if Mark kissed her – the kind of kiss that's more than a peck on the lips – her immediate thought was 'Oh no! He wants sex and I'm not feeling like it! I better close it down now so he doesn't get the wrong idea.' She had started to wear more to bed, and avoided any conversations about sex, mostly as she felt awkward, or wanted to sidestep a row.

Because of this, they had far less sexual stimuli in their life than they had before. They had stopped kissing passionately unless it was part of sex, and she didn't let Mark run his hands over her body in bed when they woke up like he used to, as she could feel him getting hard and this made her worry. Mark picked up on all of this and stopped touching Amy in this way or telling her he fancied her, as it was met with this reaction.

Amy and Mark had young children and were pretty much always exhausted. By the time they had put the kids to bed, tidied up, cooked dinner and got everything ready for the next day, they were shattered and keen to go to sleep. If they did try to have sex at these times, Amy found herself distracted by thoughts of 'have I got everything ready for the kids tomorrow?' or 'I have to be up in six hours', which made it hard for her to experience much arousal and desire. Sometimes she'd be happy to have sex anyway, more for Mark's pleasure than hers (and also as she felt it was unkind to turn him down once he'd got turned on), and these more perfunctory sexual experiences were lacking in pleasure for her. Mark would come and then they would go to sleep, without even discussing her pleasure or satisfaction.

Amy noticed that she did feel the sensation of arousal in her genitals every once in a while, when there was a sex scene on TV, or when she was reading a book with some hot sex in it. The problem, she said, was that it felt difficult to translate this into action with Mark, as she didn't always know what to say, or it would happen at times when the kids were awake, or she was alone. Sometimes she would choose to masturbate instead of approaching Mark, either because it was more convenient, quicker, or because her pleasure was more guaranteed, without any of the pressure of pleasing him.

Over time, they had sex less and less, and it became a bit of a sore subject. The less sex they had, the more awkward it felt to get started and the more pressure there was for it to go well and for it to be more about Mark's pleasure and preferences than Amy's. Amy started to avoid sexual stimuli more, as the longer the gaps between them having sex became, the more pressure there was for a passionate kiss to turn into more.

Amy and Mark are, in many ways, a very typical couple. At this stage, my hope is that, in this example, you can spot all of the different aspects of the picture that we have discussed in each chapter so far and how they are impacting on their sex life.

Which of the following did you notice in the example of Amy and Mark?

- ✪ What's normal about Amy's experience of desire in relation to what you have learned so far?

- ✪ Sex-positive sex education and early learning for women about sex, gender politics and appeasing others

- ✪ The impact of the orgasm gap and female sexual pleasure on desire

- ✪ The expectation of what sex looks like, men's desire and sexual scripts around how sex should be

- Their motivations for sex and why this matters

- Myths around the ease of spontaneous sex, and around three-times-a-week sex

- Relationship dynamics and sex communication, initiation, having children, sexual currency, priorities and time together

- The role of attention, distraction and negative thoughts

- The unhelpful use of labels

- The role of learning and incentive on sex

- Reductions in sexual currency

- Approach or avoidance motivations for sex

- Predictability, novelty and pressure

So what can Amy and Mark do about it?

Well, Amy and Mark can make changes related to any of the points above, or any of the factors we've discussed in this book so far. As I mentioned at the very start of the book, a significant change for some couples can come from understanding things differently, and an adjustment in, for example, understanding responsive desire and increasing sexual currency is all that's needed. For others, changes across several areas are needed, and may have to happen for them to break relationship habits and find a new way forward that suits desire much better. In therapy, I would probably target every area identified in a systematic way, making sure that I'm doing so in a way where couples see changes quickly, to help them stay motivated to do things differently. For the purpose of Amy and Mark just now, let's use Basson's model as a framework for mapping out where the room for change is in their sex life moving forward. At the end of this chapter I'll encourage you to develop a similar understanding for yourself and see if there are any changes you feel could be useful in your own sex life. And, in Part Three, we'll be taking those ideas forward.

Moving forward

Amy's new understanding of desire would hopefully mean that she would be feeling more receptive to or willing to seek out sexual stimuli, though it's important to note that she would need to be feeling emotionally intimate as a foundation (so it would be useful for her to reflect on how their relationship is going generally). She would also need to feel confident that this receptivity wouldn't always be positioned as the green light for sex.

As a couple, they would benefit from resurrecting the things she enjoys but doesn't let Mark do for fear of it having to turn into more. This might be about reinstating passionate kissing for kissing's sake, or massage, allowing Mark to touch her in bed in the mornings again, or always wearing little to bed, not just when she feels like sex. This would bring a change in the sexual currency between them.

In fact, if I were seeing them for therapy, I'd recommend they have a period of a few weeks where they complete the 'sexual currency overload' exercise (at the end of Chapter 5), so that they can see first-hand what difference it makes to desire if they flood their relationship with sexual stimuli, without pressure. An exercise like this gives couples an opportunity to get reacquainted with flirting, reinstating or strengthening the relationship between them as a sexual one, creating more of an association of your partner as a sexual being, and many more opportunities to trigger desire. Again, for this to be useful for their sex life, Mark would need to commit to these things not needing to lead anywhere so that there is truly no pressure and that there is no expectation that either of them should feel desire. Many couples find that making this subtle change immediately starts to improve their sexual satisfaction, even in the absence of sex. For example, one of Mark's reasons for having sex was to feel wanted, and this was why he was so concerned about Amy's avoidance. Imagine the effect it would have on Mark to have Amy sending him suggestive texts or flirting with him throughout the day.

Amy and Mark might want to try making more time together to really connect without the kids, both emotionally and physically. This doesn't need to be outside their home, if a babysitter is out of reach. It could involve an evening of making dinner for each other, for example, talking without the distraction of TV or devices, having a bath together, or going to bed early to chat naked under the covers. Even better if they can make some time for self-expanding activities, such as learning a new skill together, trying a new sport or going somewhere different and fun. Creating space for physical intimacy that might trigger desire is also important if we want to kickstart our responsive desire, so they might want to kiss, lie naked in bed together and talk, or have an evening once a fortnight where they give each other a massage. Remember that arousal and desire might need to be triggered. Spending time together might not be enough without more physical / sexual triggers.

Ultimately, Mark and Amy need to decide what priority sex should have and treat it as such, carving out regular time and space between them to have more triggers of desire without pressure for it to lead to more. Often I get asked what I think about scheduling sex as a strategy for couples in long-term relationships. The answer is that scheduling sex is rarely a good idea, as it creates pressure to have to feel/do something, but scheduling physical intimacy for the sake of physical intimacy is always a good idea, as it is both enjoyable in its own right, keeps this part of a relationship high on the priority list and provides the perfect environment for responsive desire.

Amy might identify that she would like to feel more comfortable with her body and might work on this by avoiding any media or social media that portrays unrealistic or 'perfect' body shapes. She might also find ways to reduce her stress levels more generally. They are both shattered, and they may find that, if bedtime is really the only time they can schedule physical intimacy, they might want to move their bedtime thirty minutes earlier, in the hope of reducing their overall tiredness. Even better still, spend this time together as soon as the kids are asleep, rather than last thing at night. Amy struggles with distraction, and negative thoughts are a big feature of their current sex life. She would benefit from starting a mindfulness practice outside of sex, with the aim of moving it into sex in time, as well as reducing her general stress levels.

Amy is carrying all the psychological burden of the household chores and family admin tasks, without this ever having been discussed and agreed by both of them. They could decide to share this more equally so that Amy doesn't find herself going to bed worrying about all the tasks that need to be completed for the kids the next day, knowing that, if she doesn't do it, no one will. It's important for Mark to understand that this is one of her barriers to desire, even if it wouldn't be to him. In some ways, this is where gendered scripts of responsibility might need to be spelled out as operating differently for women and men.

Ideally, Amy should move towards a belief that it's not acceptable for Mark to enjoy sex more than her, and to not accept sex with low reward every time as the status quo. Amy has never felt confident asking for what she wants during sex and, especially now, her enjoyment is really important. Can Mark make her come easily? Does he know how? If this is not the case, Amy needs to teach him, and Mark needs to be committed to learning. Amy and Mark would benefit from having equal amounts of sex that prioritize Mark's pleasure (like vaginal penetration), and Amy's (like oral sex), rather than their sex life always following a set and predictable pattern ending in penetrative vaginal sex. It's important that they consider the role of predictability and novelty in their sexual expression, in how their sex looks and the freedom they both have for sexual expression of different types.

Amy is sometimes having sex for avoidance reasons, meaning she is having sex to avoid conflict rather than because she wants to, or for Mark's pleasure. Amy's long-term desire would benefit from no longer continuing to have sex for these reasons. If Mark wants to be sexual and Amy doesn't feel 'receptive' to seeing if her arousal can be triggered, then they would benefit from talking more about what's behind Mark's motivations for sex on that day and whether there are any other ways it can be met. Amy could use that opportunity to reassure Mark if he's feeling insecure.

We could go on. But hopefully you can see that there are lots of ways Amy and Mark can start to turn this around now that they understand desire better. I've worked with hundreds of couples over the years who have made huge changes to their sex lives by first understanding this then making practical changes to how they are sexual together. A small change in any area usually has a positive impact, but a handful of changes, like those suggested above, can make a massive impact to a couple's sex life over time.

So where are you at? Consider the points below to reflect on this before we move on to Part Three.

- Prior to reading this book, how much did you subscribe to the belief that you should be feeling spontaneous sexual desire (rate it as a percentage, if you like, with 100% being that you completely believed it)?

- How did this belief impact on your willingness to be receptive to sexual stimuli in the way it did for some of the women in the examples?

- What have you found yourself doing/not doing not to give your partner the 'wrong idea' in response to this?

- What has your partner stopped doing over time as a result?

- What would be the effect on your sex life if you started to be more willing to trigger arousal and desire? (note: if you are going to do this, have a discussion with your partner about the importance of there needing to be no pressure for this to turn into more)

My hope is that your understanding of how desire might work for you is different now this book has provided you with some ideas about how desire is given the opportunity to flourish, or is inhibited, in your own sex life.

Generally, with most areas of our life where we want to create change, it can be useful to first understand what's going on and then to put a plan in place that we know will undermine what's keeping us stuck. Desire is no different. For some people, simply hearing about how desire works *is* the quick fix, as knowing they are normal and understanding their body are all they need to take the stress of the situation away or know how to action it. For others, the additional step of making a plan to undermine any previously less helpful patterns, as outlined in the actions Amy and Mark could take above, will take you closer to a more rewarding sex life.

If you're interested, it can be really helpful to start building up your own personalized visual picture of how desire features in your sex life, including ideas from everything you've read so far. The key features should include: your sexual history, societal messages, the context of your relationship and what's happening in your mind, as well as aspects from the circular model presented in this chapter, such as receptivity, sexual stimuli, barriers to desire and the effects of positive or negative rewards. Doing this will help you identify what you can do to create positive change in your sex life, should you feel (as is the case with most of us) that your sex life has room for improvement.

There is no doubt that we all have our own individual relationship with sex, which is based on our unique histories, contexts and life experiences up until this point, and that these influence our desire. It's also true that these experiences play out consciously and unconsciously in what's going on in our minds and relationships. But it doesn't stop there. Desire is a fluid entity that is cultivated or extinguished minute by minute, day by day, between us and a partner, based on how we nurture it. Defining our and our partner's desire as fixed, static and not amenable to change, based on our past experiences of it, is the first obstacle we create to long-term sexual satisfaction, as it forms a perception that nothing we do or say makes a difference and that it's a problem with us. Framing desire in this way not only stops us from making any effort to guide our sex life in the way we want it to go, but it prevents us from being curious to learn anything about how desire *actually works*.

Take-home messages from this chapter

- ⮑ Women's' desire is more often *responsive* rather than *spontaneous* in long-term relationships

- ⮑ Waiting for sexual desire before being receptive to sexual stimuli, like a touch, a kiss or being naked together, might result in less and less sexual contact over time

- ⮑ Societal messages tell us the opposite (based largely on an outdated and male-focused model of sexual response), but this makes us feel bad, as we wonder what is wrong with us and our relationships

- ⮑ Our partners wonder too, and they might wonder why, take it personally, or evaluate it as a problem

- ⮑ This can lead to conflict at worst, awkwardness at best, and make sex the 'elephant in the room' or a sore point in our relationship.

- ⮑ We might try to avoid conflict by trying not to give our partners the wrong idea by being less receptive to sexual stimuli or by closing down any advances by our partners by giving verbal or non-verbal clues of 'not interested'

- ⮑ Women's sexual desire is very easily triggered, but we don't get to see or benefit from this, as we stop any chances of desire emerging with the above strategies

- ⮑ Kissing, touching and other flirtation falls more and more off the agenda and we can get out of sync with what works to turn each other on, or things that would have been considered sexual stimuli in the first few years of our relationship become so infrequent that we feel odd doing it together, and it becomes like a big neon sign over both of us, saying 'sex is on the agenda' (which is, of course, offputting)

- ⮑ When we feel pressure to feel desire, such as on a weekend away, this acts as a psychological barrier which, paradoxically, inhibits desire

- ⮑ Understanding how desire works and mapping out ways to encourage it to thrive based on these understandings is the key

Exercise:
Reflection – sexual stimuli, hot or not?

Construct a list like Amy's from earlier in this chapter. Try to come up with something your partner does that doesn't necessarily work, something that does and which you want them to keep doing, and something you've never mentioned but you'd be keen for them to try at some point in the future. It's good to be honest, but please be careful how you phrase things that could be taken personally or construed by your partner as them not being good enough. For example, Amy could say to Mark: 'I can't stand it when you grab my boobs out of the blue – it's awful!' Instead, she might say: 'I sometimes find sensitive areas like my breasts are not the best place to touch first – it can feel a bit too much! I really like it when you touch me around my shoulders and neck first.' If you've been together a long time and you've never discussed these things, do be aware that it can feel hurtful to be told many years in that you've never liked something that your partner has been doing.

What would make this exercise even more effective would be to explain it to your partner and have them construct their own list, to give you some insight also.

Take time together to share your lists and remember the principles of:

1) Listening well

2) Not ridiculing each other's lists

3) Making an attempt to sidestep well-practised and familiar arguments about it

4) Being careful with the words you use: go gently

Trying it out – an experiment in kickstarting desire

This is an experiment with the circular model alone, to see what you notice in your body. Find some time to be alone privately and choose a film or book that you know has sex scenes in it, erotic literature or audio stories or porn you feel comfortable watching. Notice the sensations you feel in your body, particularly in your genitals. If you don't notice anything, ask yourself – is the scene you are watching/reading arousing to you or is it a turn-off? If the scene is arousing but you are not noticing any sensation, could there be any particular psychological, situational or physical barriers getting in the way (e.g. tiredness, stress, worry about being interrupted, feeling shame about what turns you on, etc.). Try this several times. It's likely that you will experience genital arousal, and this might turn into psychological desire. What does this tell you about what you might need more of in your own sex life? What does it tell you about how the circular model fits for you? What would happen if you started to build more of these cues into your own life, day to day, or as part of investing in spending some time fantasizing from time to time?

Three

How to Futureproof Your Sex Life, for Life

8

What next?

In Part One I set the scene for the reasons women's sexuality has the place that it does in history, culture, politics and science. We understood the importance of understanding our preferences and our anatomy and reflected on how all the gaps we currently have in our sex lives or in our understanding of sex inhibit, or misrepresent, women's sexual desire.

In Part Two, I took you through the impact that society has had on how we socialize women to be sexually, but also the impact of how we teach women to see their bodies and their place in society more widely. We looked at the impact of relationship dynamics, communication and the meaning of sex, as well as the impact of our brains in processing our past history, our thoughts and our attention. We learned about models of desire that women often feel more aptly help them conceptualize their desire, and how these models, based more accurately on the science of desire, make sense of the experience of large numbers of women sitting at home waiting to feel something that is unlikely to come.

By now, my hope is that you feel what you've read so far has connected you with your experience of your sexuality in a way you haven't ever considered before. When I started writing this book, I wanted it to be the book that I wanted all women to read, given that my clinics were full of women thinking they were broken when they were not; women and couples feeling powerless to resolve issues of conflict related to sex, even when their relationships were otherwise strong. For years I've imagined the impact of some of this information being known on a wider scale than it currently is, and the impact this could have on people's life satisfaction and relationships, as well as their sex lives. In this final part of the book my aim is to encourage you to look forwards, both at how you might create change based on what you've learned, and how you might futureproof your sex life by steering it in the direction you want, rather than letting it drift somewhere you don't.

How does change happen?

Change can happen in a number of ways. The new understanding you have gained might be the only change you need, and you might now respond and react to your sex life in a few key ways which are low in effort but have a large impact on your sexual satisfaction. For some people and relationships, small changes have far-reaching consequences. Alternatively, perhaps you are seeing things differently but there is a bit more work that needs to be put in for you to feel you will really see change. The latter might be especially likely if you have found yourself falling into any of the less helpful habits we've spoken about, and many of the exercises you have already completed will be the facilitators of a change in this, to start things moving in another direction.

In this chapter I'm going to be helping you think through how you put this plan into action and how you might get someone else on board with this idea. The thing about sex, of course, is that it often involves more than one person, and sometimes it doesn't matter how much our perception or understanding changes – if that other person is not on the same page, they are unable to jump on our sexual revolution bandwagon.

Getting partners on board

When it comes to partners, the simplest thing you could do is get them to read this book. Or, at the very least, ask them to read the bits that made the most sense or had the biggest impact on you. In the absence of this, of if they read it and still feel cautious, here are my top tips for getting them onboard in a way that can help you make changes:

1) State what you feel the impact of making changes might be

2) Talk thought the effect you feel this will have on you/them/the relationship

3) Speculate that it must be tough for them to hear facts and ideas that contradict all they've understood about sex so far in life, especially since the current messages feel like they are in their favour

4) Suggest that, although a change in the way you think of or 'do' sex might feel like it's moving away from their preferences in favour of yours, it's actually benefitting you both, as it's future-proofing your sex life over time

5) Tell them they don't have to believe that everything in this book, or that you're telling them, is true, but just to agree to suspend judgement to test it out, with the intention of gathering evidence to see whether it works

Here's an example of how this conversation might go, between Jamilia and Adam.

Jamilia: Hey! I've been meaning to tell you about this book that I've been reading, all about sex and women's sex lives. It's got some shocking stuff in there about the fact that women's sex lives in heterosexual sex have always been sidelined in favour of men's. You know, 'cos of the patriarchy and everything, and that, actually, although there are tons of women feeling like there's something wrong with their desire, there's actually nothing wrong with their desire except the way in which they've been doing sex, and the way they've been understanding desire and stuff. It's got me really thinking about our sex life and that we should do something different.

Adam: What's wrong with our sex life?

Jamelia: Well, nothing major. You know it's great when we do it, but I know you always feel like you want it more than me, and I always feel like there's, you know, pressure for me to feel like it, and I just think it could be better, you know?

Adam: Erm . . . I've never heard you say this before . . .

Jamelia: To be honest, I've never said anything as I've always thought there was something wrong with me, as in every relationship I've had I feel really into sex for the first few months or year and then I just start to feel really uninterested. Since I've read this book, I've been thinking that the influence of worrying about how I look all the time, or how my family talked about sex being really dirty, is probably coming into it, but now I've found out that this experience of desire is normal, and that I – we – can do something different about it. I think it would be great? Don't you?

Adam: I just thought it was all right as it was, to be honest, but I suppose it has been the thing we've rowed most about.

Jamelia: Yeah. I just keep thinking what it would be like to get out of that cycle of you going on about sex like it's my duty and me feeling pressured to do it and then us both getting all stressed and narky about it. I think if we did this, we might both feel a bit more equal and relaxed about it, you know? And also it might mean that we get to feel even more connected in that way. I think it would be really good for us. I'd like it if I thought about and felt like sex more, you know? It would make me feel normal and that we were really solid.

Adam: I'd really like that too, actually. I do sometimes wish I felt like I wasn't always the one bringing it up, as it sometimes makes me feel like you don't want me, or you're not that into it. What kinds of things are in this book, then?

Jamelia: Oh, it's probably best if you read it, but there's stuff around the fact that women's desire is more responsive than spontaneous – it needs triggering rather than being something that just happens – but that as we often expect desire to come first, we don't try and trigger it but just wait until it happens, which it often doesn't. There's also stuff about how sex between men and women isn't really the type of sex physically that works best for women, and that this leads to sex carrying less pleasure than it could, oh – and stuff around how the best type of sex life is one with loads of variety and not always ending in penis-in-vagina sex as, like, the 'main course' of sex.

Adam: That sounds drastic and a bit weird.

Jamelia: Okay . . . well, I'm not sure we really need you to believe it all, actually . . . and I know it must be hard as, without either of us even realizing it, sex might have been skewed towards the types of sex that fit your preferences and anatomy over mine, so it's bound to sound less appealing to you. But if you agree that if we could feel more equal and argue less about sex, perhaps you can suspend your judgement for a few months and see it as a bit of an experiment, then decide what you make of it? You will have to really try, though; I can't do it on my own, as then it just won't work. It's a two-person job. What do you think? Shall we do it?!?

Adam: Okay. I'll reserve judgement. Let's give it a go.

Jamelia employed points 1–5 in her conversation with Adam (though, unfortunately, if he's now read the book, he's also probably realized that was what she was doing). She stayed away from any heavy critique of their sex lives, instead selling a picture of what it would be like if it were different. She focuses not on changing his understanding at this stage (as the force is strong when it comes to social scripts and societal norms), but instead just asks for his participation in a trial of doing things differently. All Jamelia needs is Adam's commitment to try to be an active participant and to let the changes that happen as a result of their actions influence his understanding and potentially make a permanent change in how he sees things.

In my clinical work, if I'm working with a heterosexual couple, it can sometimes be the case that the male partner struggles to get on board with all the ideas we've talked about, and another small gap opens up, where the female partner suddenly feels understood and revitalized, can see what might be the impact of them doing things differently, and is galvanized into action. He, on the other hand, can sometimes find this new way of relating to sex and desire hard to grasp, mainly as if it doesn't fit his experience (for example, he is someone with high levels of spontaneous desire, and is really wedded to an idea that this is preferable, 'right' and 'normal'). It's also fair to say that, although not a conscious resistance, the movement of the location of the problem in his mind from 'there's something wrong with her sex drive', which affects me, to 'as a couple we need to manage our sex lives differently to keep us both interested and fulfilled' can be a hard move to make. After all, the male partner may have started the process feeling like he had no problem, and he's there to support someone else, and he ends the process understanding the role that he is playing, unknowingly, is both causing and maintaining it. He is also now an active agent required to put in 'work'. Saying all of this, I have worked with many men who at first felt quite resistant, but were happy to experiment with making some changes to test out these ideas, who experienced this process as revelatory and hugely rewarding once they invested in it.

For same-sex couples, it can be the same scenario, where one person experiences high levels of spontaneous desire, and one doesn't, but in my experience the process of social and cultural learning that women share means that, when I talk through these things with two women, they can often both get on board with it, even if one of them has a slightly different experience than the other.

What do you stand to lose or gain?

At this point I'd also suggest that it might be worth taking a moment to reflect on the future trajectory of your sex life, should you decide not to take any action. Consider how things are now and how long you've been together. Consider any life challenges you might have coming your way (such as becoming parents, ill health, ageing and body changes). Now imagine what the sex life you have now might be like in five years, ten years, twenty years, based on what you've learned. Ask yourself the following questions about your current (or future) sex life trajectory:

- What would it be like if the current pattern we have beds in even more or is amplified over time?

- How essential do I feel mutual pleasure, sexual adventure and sexual fulfilment are to both of us for long-term sexual satisfaction?

- How has my sexuality evolved in the past fifteen years? Is my current sex life a fertile ground to allow it to evolve this much again over the next fifteen? Or might it by stifled by habit, expectation and routine?

- How able will we be to withstand the impact of significant life changes on our sex life?

- How able will we be to negotiate mutually satisfying change when we need to?

- If something happened which meant we could no longer have sex in the way we currently do, what impact would this have on our relationship satisfaction?

These questions are a starting point for you to consider your sex life now but also to think realistically about where it's headed in its current form. Our sexuality is a lifelong journey for all of us, and it changes as a result of changes in identity, in our circumstances, in perspective and in our body. The contexts of our sexual relationships need to be able to allow room for this growth and adaptation, so that each of us can experience more sexual satisfaction as we age, not less.

Working on your own sexuality

Given that our sexuality is a lifelong journey, it's also worth noting that it's a journey that we are in control of. Yes, the influences of our lives so far, including social learning, shame, unwanted or abusive sexual experiences, may have steered it to places we are not totally happy with thus far, but, from here on in, it's up to us to create situations and contexts which amplify our sexual confidence and facilitate our sexual exploration in a way which benefits the sex life we have with others. We have covered how the relationship we have with our sexual selves is a key part of how we relate to sex with others, and this relationship is something we all have direct control over.

Women who masturbate have higher levels of sexual satisfaction than women who don't.[1] Not only does masturbation help us explore what we like without the pressure of someone else's preferences, it allows us to push boundaries privately, explore a rich fantasy or erotica world, and have positive, rewarding sexual experiences that boost our desire and keep sex in the forefront of our minds. There's also research to suggest that women who masturbate more frequently show greater concordance.[2]

There is no doubt that masturbation is a great way to get comfortable and continually evolve and build positive association with our sexuality, but our sexuality is so much more than the physical, and exploring our sexual self in ANY way can be useful. Whether it's through art, reading, music, by talking with friends, in the way you dress, through dancing – there are many ways we can practise engaging with our sexual selves in a way that builds confidence with who we are and what we need.

Sexual confidence is just one aspect of who we are, but if we're struggling with it, it can really impact on our sex lives with others. Focusing on developing our own sexuality and sexual confidence is known to be good for long-term desire.[3] It's important to remember that we're all on a journey with this and no one has it totally sorted or feels crazy confident all of the time. Most of us just need to work out the contexts in our life that build or knock our confidence (in sex, in relationships, with friends, with work, on social media) and pay attention to how they do this, then act accordingly.

- What contexts increase your sexual confidence and how accessible are they to you right now?

- What things do you feel you need to work on or connect with alone to benefit your sexuality with others?

- What aspects of your sexuality would you like to invest in that you currently don't?

If there are things you've identified that would make a difference to how you feel about sex or your sexuality, and ways you feel you could invest in this part of yourself outside of your relationship, then this is something to consider as part of investing in your sex life in the long term.

Maximizing success – where do you want to go?

One of the factors that will give you the most chances of success with futureproofing your sex life (alongside new understandings and having a shared commitment to making it happen) is having a clear co-constructed idea of where you want to go. This is the same in face-to-face sex therapy, and I never start off a piece of work with an individual or a couple without having the final destination clearly and explicitly mapped out. There are several reasons for this: knowing where you are going provides an indication to all involved about the key steps needed to get there; starting off talking about where you want to be creates a shared vision that makes you feel more connected with each other and the plan; and talking about the ideal rather than the problematic version of your sex life is what psychologists call 'problem-free talk', and creates hope and optimism that benefits your journey.[4] It also provides a much-needed *different* type of conversation about sex, which is especially useful if the same conversations about sex – 'You always do this, you never do that, etc., etc.' – happen so regularly that you can predict who will start it, who will say what and when, who will get defensive, who will get angry and what format the unsatisfactory conclusion would take. In fact, the whole point of therapy, especially with couples, is to have a different experience of talking about something which is very familiar to you both. After all, if the same conversations were helpful, people wouldn't be stuck with them in the first place.

I often explain to clients that a good therapist is like a black cab driver (sorry, Uber). When you get in the cab, they should have no opinion on where you go, only the knowledge, means and expertise to get you there in the most efficient and effective way. It's very common in therapy for people to be extremely adept at explaining to you where they don't want to go. Destinations like 'I just don't want to feel like this any more', 'I want him to stop going on about it', 'I don't want our sex life to be like this', are really common ones for people to offer up in response to the question of where they want to be by the end of the work. The thing is, these answers give no clue about where they want to go, just where they don't want to go. They are the equivalent of me getting in a black cab and saying, 'I don't want to go to St Paul's Cathedral. It makes me feel rubbish,' A bad black cab driver would say, 'Okay, great' and just start driving aimlessly around London, avoiding St Paul's and hoping they would stumble on the right place eventually. A slightly more effective driver might think, 'Okay, they don't want St Paul's, so I'll take them to another cathedral? Westminster Abbey it is,' and perhaps drive them to a similar location (this is an example of where the bias of the cab driver comes in – they have guessed it's another cathedral the person wants but, of course, this is just their perspective and they could well be wrong). A good black cab driver would say, 'Okay, I understand you don't want to go to St Paul's, but where is it exactly that you do want to go?' Good therapy is a bit like this, but the problem is that we are socially conditioned through the media to believe that therapy is all about talking about what's going wrong rather than what you would like to be happening instead, so those alternative destinations often need lots of encouragement in the early sessions in order to develop them fully.

I especially enjoy spending time with individuals or couples at the start of our work talking not just about where they want to go (and reaching a destination that suits both of them) but also what the impact of getting to their destination will be on them individually, and the relationship. This is useful as a) their goals are usually very achievable and it's useful to have a hopeful conversation, bringing to life this more satisfying future sex life, especially if they've been worrying about it for some time, and b) asking why this destination is important to them and what difference it will make to get there tells us all a great deal about what's really important and why. This is often the start of the real work, as it may be a level of depth to talking about sex that's never been reached by them before, as often people get stuck at the same surface-level gripes about things, such as frequency of sex, for example, with the same unsatisfactory outcomes.

Let's use these same therapy concepts to consider how you can maximize success to get the sex life you want moving forward. It doesn't matter if your sex life feels desperately broken, or if it's wonderfully satisfying and you just want to take time to prioritize and nurture it. In either scenario a conversation following the below structure will be helpful.

Picking your moment

The best time to have a conversation about sex is when you're feeling connected, close and content. Starting from a place of irritation, anger or distance is not an inherently bad place to speak from but might make it more challenging for either of you to feel open, honest and transparent about how you feel and to listen and really hear what someone else thinks. Sometimes people can feel as though raising things you'd like to be different at a time when things are going really well – such as on a really fun weekend away together – is a bad idea, as it would 'rock the boat' and ruin an otherwise great time. This is especially true for those whose concerns about sex might be connected to a history of resentment or arguments, as opposed to those who have no major concerns but want to create space in their sex life for expansion and growth. But it's important to remember that a good conversation, where you both feel heard and you share ideas of where you want to go, could be a very positive experience and make an already blissful time away even better. Similarly, talking about things you want to be different does not have to mean you spend an hour talking about how much you hate St Paul's. You can spend that hour talking about all the places in London you love to go and you miss visiting instead. The latter conversation in relation to your sex life will generally leave both of you feeling much more positive than the former, even though you're essentially talking about the exact same thing.

How to have this conversation

There are four key aspects to this conversation that you can use as guiding principles.

1. What you appreciate / what you used to appreciate; state that you miss / want it

2. What you'd like to build on / where you'd like things to go

3. What difference you think it would make to you / the relationship if you got there

4. Inviting their perspective and response to this and being able to listen and really hear it

This is a slightly different version of the conversation Jamelia and Adam had earlier, building on the concept of the destination more clearly. Here's where their conversation got to:

> **Jamelia:** I've been thinking about our sex life and how it's changed a bit recently and I was remembering all the things I used to love about it that we don't do so much of any more. Like, do you remember when we used to get all excited about having time together to have sex? You used to send me texts throughout the day telling me how much you fancied me and all the things you were thinking of doing. I used to love that.

Adam: Oh yeah, I miss that too. But I also miss how much you used to seem into me, like knowing that you were looking forward to it as much as me, and that you couldn't wait to see me.

Jamelia: Do you? Oh, I didn't realize . . . And when we spent time together I used to feel like you really took your time on me, like really spending time being close, kissing, touching me all over my body and stuff. We used to have much longer, more time to really enjoy it. I miss that, as it feels like we don't take the time as much any more? I was thinking that it feels a bit harder to be like that now we're living together. There's not really an opportunity to miss each other and get excited about seeing each other in that way, plus we've often got other things to do, so sex takes a bit of a back seat.

Adam: Yes, I think you're right. I miss that too, but I suppose I often do rush it a bit more now, as I don't feel like you're as into it as you were back then, so I feel like I'm doing you a favour by making it quicker and getting to the point.

Jamelia: Oh, really? That's ironic! It would be great if we could bring those days back again, don't you think? Like, not always or every time we have sex, as I know things are different in our life now, but if we could have the odd time, like once a month, where we made a bit of a deal of it and got each other excited about it over the course of the day. I'd like to have that anticipation back. I think it would make me feel more into it, which might make you feel like I was more into it and into you?

Adam: Yes, that sounds good. I just haven't been doing those things, as I thought you'd feel like I was harassing you about it. I'd

> love it if it was you that suggested it as well, so I don't always feel like it's up to me and you're just going along with it?
>
> **Jamelia**: Okay, let's do that. I think it will really bring back some excitement into our sex life and make us feel close again. I also think that having sex like that would really be good for my desire.

The problem and the solution to having the sex life that you want lies between you and the person (or people) you are having sex with, and in many ways this is both the curse and the joy of sex. We've spoken so far in this book about all the ways that you relate to sex and how these things impact your sex life, but it would be a huge omission to assume that you can make these changes without bringing who-ever you're having sex with on board with you. The more of these types of conversations you have, the more chance there is that you can move towards a sex life that allows you space for satisfaction, pleasure and desire, but also sets the scene for a sex life that will allow space to grow, adapt and expand.

Take-home messages from this chapter

- ➲ Making changes based on your new understanding can come from understanding things differently, or doing things differently

- ➲ Doing things differently works best with the understanding and commitment of whoever else is involved

- ➲ Making changes such as the ones in this book goes against the grain of how we've been brought up to think about sex and can be challenging

- ⮑ Partners might find this hard to get on board with, but they need to be open to the idea of testing this out (rather than being fully sold on it immediately)

- ⮑ Not doing anything is also doing something, as your sex life is already on a trajectory that will lead to a destination eventually, whether that destination is your preferred one or not

- ⮑ Investing in your own sexuality is a crucial part of this journey and is about much more than masturbation

- ⮑ Being clear about the destination you both want to go to, and what difference you feel this would make, makes getting there easier

9

Futureproof your sex life, for life

G iven everything we've covered in this book so far, it should come as no surprise to you that your sex life (as well as your sexual desire) will not follow a fixed, predictable or set trajectory from here on in. That is not to say that there cannot be a general 'up trend' in your sexual satisfaction from now until you take your last breath – I believe there can. But, rather, this general increase in satisfaction that you can achieve with *purposeful intention and action*, as I've described in this book, will see peaks and troughs, ups and downs and ebbs and flows, as you, your body, your mind and your relationship adapt to challenges and circumstances that come your way. It is the foundations that you put in place for your sex life, the beliefs you have about your sex life, and the way you respond and communicate about these challenges that will result in long-term sexual satisfaction.

In this final chapter we will consider what constitutes a 'good' sex life over time and work out what this means for you. We will reflect on the kinds of life events that can result in this ebb and flow and necessitate adaptation. We will look at what the research tells us are the behaviours and qualities associated with long-term sexual satisfaction and how you can apply these to your own sex life in a tailored and convenient way. Crucially, given that a good sex life for many couples isn't accidental, we'll look at the actions and strategies you can put in place to futureproof your sex life, for life.

What do we mean by a good sex life?

Sometimes, when people talk about a good sex life they use it as a synonym for frequency. Evaluating a sex life on the basis of frequency is one of the greatest red herrings we have at our disposal as a society when it comes to 'good sex'. Frequency tells us nothing about connection, pleasure, variety, intimacy, adventure, passion, expression or novelty. It tells us that sex is happening, yes. But as we've learned so far, if sex is happening frequently but the sex that is happening is lacking in emotional or physical reward, it's usually not only not good sex but it's potentially lowering our desire and sexual satisfaction slowly but surely over time.

So, what is the definition of good sex? Well, the truth is no one can define that but you, but I can offer you some ideas to help your thinking. You'll remember early on in this book we talked about your 'conditions for good sex'. This was a guide to considering how your psychological arousal, physical touch and being-in-the-moment are important to you to allow you to really enjoy sex. It's likely that a possible definition of good sex for you is not about frequency but about the presence or absence of these things. My hope is that this book may have given you the rationale and the confidence to seek out or insist on these conditions moving forwards, even if cultural/ religious/gendered restrictions based on societal messages have held you back from doing so thus far.

Establishing what good sex means for you might also be understanding the function of sex for you and in your relationships and working out if the original motivation you had for sex is being met when you have it. If you have sex to feel close, for example, and you find your partner distant or absorbed in their own pleasure and body in a way that makes you feel disconnected from them, perhaps this might not feel like 'good sex' to you, even if it looks on the surface like it's meeting your conditions. Hopefully, you have spent some time reflecting on the function that sex serves in your life and relationship and you are closer than you have been before to understanding this. Crucially, if you have had this discussion with a partner, you will also have a greater understanding of your partner's motivations for sex, which may have given you a totally different perspective on what's important to them and why.

Good sex for you might mean changing the sexual script in your relationship, including more novelty, more variety and more pleasure from non-penetrative sex acts than you've ever had before. As you now know, such a change is not just about more consistent pleasure for women (though it definitely leads to it), but rather a way to make sex more playful, less boring and keep desire alive over time.

Lastly, good sex for you might mean having less sex than you do now but feeling connected sexually in other ways (using sexual currency) and having the confidence to know this is something that you don't need to worry about. Sex once a year can be just the ticket if it's the kind of sex that meets both of your needs and makes you feel alive.

I'd like you to reflect on all we've covered in this book so far, to work out what your definition of 'good sex' at this moment in time is. Consider your 'conditions' triangle, the shackles of social scripts and the constraining beliefs about sex we've talked about, aspects of your relationship more widely, the habits you've got into that you'd like to break free of, the impact of your mind on sex, the emphasis on your pleasure and your new-found understanding of how desire works.

How important is frequency? How important is connection? Intimacy? Pleasure? Variety? Equality? Passion? Trust? Exploration? If you can, make a note somewhere detailing the definition of good sex for you at this point in your life. Try to be as thorough as you can be, and if you feel able and have one at the moment, ask your partner to do the same. Knowing the key aspects of each other's version of a 'good' sex life right now is a crucial part of futureproofing your sex life over time, as it allows you to navigate your sex life around what's important, rather than an arbitrary societal yardstick, such as frequency.

What does the science say about what makes sex good in the long term?

Now that you've worked this out for yourself, let's also look at what science tells us about sexual satisfaction in long-term relationships. Recent ground-breaking research tells us that there are several qualities of sex lives that are associated with couples who report 'good sex', and they are not necessarily the ones you'd think. Knowing about these can help you foster them or aspire to do more of them to see what difference they can make for you.

Responsiveness

'Communal giving' is a term used to describe giving to others when we don't expect to receive in return[1] and 'communal strength' is a term used to describe how inclined we might be to meet the needs of a partner.[2] The basic principle of communal strength is that we place value on meeting a partner's needs for the sake of meeting their needs and not for our own personal gain. We meet needs that are within our ability/resources, and not unreasonable, and we trust that at some future point they will meet our needs in return. Sexual communal strength has been defined by Amy Muise and colleagues as the ability to be receptive to a partner's sexual needs (to have or not have sex as well as how), based on their partner's wants and preferences rather than the impact that this might have on them.[3] This might include things like agreeing to have sex when they aren't really feeling like it,* trying out things our partners are interested in, or being understanding about a partner's desire not to have sex. Research has found that, in long-term relationships, people who report higher levels of communal strength in their relationship report higher levels of sexual satisfaction and desire.[4] There is, of course, an interesting nuance here in heterosexual relationships, where gender equality intersects with sexual communal strength. For example, how does this responsiveness play out when there is a gendered script of whose pleasure is expected as a given, with weighted opinion on the expectation of men's pleasure as a priority?

It can be useful for all of us to consider how empathic we are towards our partner's needs and wants sexually, and the positive change in desire or satisfaction we both might see if we were prepared to sometimes put our partner's sexual needs before our own without expecting anything in return. Being overly fixated on your own needs, wants and preferences, as opposed to someone else's, or having a strong sense of personal sexual entitlement (dubbed 'sexual narcissism') lowers sexual satisfaction and desire for *both* partners over the course of a relationship.[5]

---

* There are limits to this. Having repeated experiences of consensual unwanted sex is not helpful for long-term sexual desire. Agreeing to have sex when you're not feeling like it in terms of sexual communal strength refers to feeling sexually neutral, but being willing to have sex from time to time, with an idea that responsive desire and enjoyment might follow rather than having sex for avoidance motivations, such as to avoid a row.

Conscientiousness

Sex researchers have moved outside the realms of sex to look at personality characteristics and how they impact on sexual satisfaction in relationships more generally. Fascinatingly, in one study published in *The Journal of Sex Research*, a personality trait found to predict sexual satisfaction was conscientiousness.[6]

Conscientiousness, typically described as being good at planning, attention to detail, being organized and dependable, is not necessarily the one personality trait of the 'Big Five' (the constructs we usually think of as defining people- the other four are openness to experience, extraversion, agreeableness and neuroticism) that you would expect to see connected with better sex. Or perhaps not until reading this book. Conscientiousness seems like a surprise due to our societal emphasis on good sex being about *spontaneity* and *passion*. However, it's likely that conscientiousness is so good for our sex lives as people who have more conscientious traits are more likely to factor in time to be intimate, to consider their partner's needs, try hard to please, remember what partners like and spend time considering setting the context and overcoming obstacles. All things which I'm sure you can see at this stage might be good for long-term desire and particularly good for scheduling emotional and physical intimacy.

Self-expanding activities

Another key influential study has added to what we know about how we spend time with our partners and the impact of this on sexual satisfaction and desire.

Research has already shown that couples who engage in activities that are exciting, inspiring or challenging are able to revisit or regenerate some of those much-sought-after early relationship feelings towards one another,[7] and Muise and her colleagues wanted to look at the impact of this on sexual desire.

They discovered that an injection of novelty and 'self-expansion' into ourselves or our relationship outside the bedroom can affect what happens within it, and that couples who spend more time doing novel, interesting and challenging activities individually or together see an improvement in their sex life as a result.[8] They found that couples who spent time on these self-expansion activities (as opposed to just time together as usual) were more likely to experience sexual desire, and more likely to have sex than couples who didn't.

Self-expanding activities could include things like going on a road trip together, learning to dance, developing a new skill together, or undertaking some kind of challenge, such as cooking a new meal from scratch or going rock climbing. These experiences mirror some of the earlier relationship dynamics when couples are still learning about each other and having novel experiences together. The rationale behind this is that self-expanding activities bring with them a change in intimacy, and new information or perspectives on a partner who might otherwise seem well known and overfamiliar. This can bring with it a resurgence or injection of desire. Hopefully, you can spot the link between this research and some of the relationship dynamics around overfamiliarity, intimacy and giving each other the scraps that we discussed in Chapter 5.

What's important to take note of is that, in this research, it was not the *time* couples spent together but *how they spent this time* that resulted in higher reported desire and sexual activity. Couples who found ways to 'excite, inspire and connect' with each other may have created some space to learn new things about themselves or each other and so created conditions of novelty, distance and excitement, akin to those early months, fanning the flames of desire. There was another crucial finding of this study: the longer sexual partners had been together, or the more pressed for time they were (think new parents), the more impact self-expansion activities such as these had on their sex lives.

What does this mean for our long-term sexual relationships? It means that, if we want to keep our sex lives hot, then perhaps it's time to prioritize making time to really connect, by having explorative and meaningful conversations with the intention of discovering new things about each other – not just about what we ate for lunch or who said what at the photocopier. For some of us, it might be as simple as looking at each other through another person's eyes, or in a different environment, such as watching our partners charm the new neighbours at a party. It might be planning an adventure together, trying something new and exhilarating, or learning something new. The bottom line is: the challenge to creating time together that involves something novel and exciting might take a bit of thought and planning but it could have some serious benefits to our sex lives.

Our experiences of desire and sexual satisfaction are complex, and there are many things adding to this picture (what's going on in our bodies, our personal relationship with sex, our relationship with our cultural and social contexts), but there is a tangible real-life value in studies such as this, which demystify what practical steps we can take to improve things when it comes to futureproofing our sex lives.

How to deal with being thrown off course

Earlier in this chapter I mentioned that, throughout the course of our sexual lives, there will be changes to our bodies, minds, relationships and circumstances that impact upon our sex lives, requiring a temporary halt, a change of course or even a total rethink as to what sex even is/looks like. These changes are normal and not necessarily to be feared. In fact, they provide us with an opportunity for novelty and recalibration.

The impact of life transitions, such as being pregnant, having young children, ill health, periods of intense stress, anxiety, physical changes, relationship stresses, ageing, moving house, grief and many more, will bring with them challenges for sex and desire. This might mean sex loses momentum for a while, becomes less satisfying, or that it falls off the agenda completely. This is normal and not something to worry about. In fact, research shows us that understanding that sexual desire ebbs and flows is a key predictor of long-term sexual satisfaction and that subscribing to this view is, in itself, a barrier to desire dropping.[9] One of the reasons for this is that it changes the interpretation we make of our partner's low desire if we attribute it to their stress levels rather than to something about us or our relationship. It also means we are more likely to make efforts to get things back on track. So, the first thing you need to do to keep your sex life good in the long term is to understand that *your sex life will go through up and downs* in response to these events, and that *this is to be expected*. In some ways, this is where the understanding of sex as a fluid and responsive *motivation*, rather than a *drive*, comes in, as it helps make sense of these changes when they happen, unlike the fixed idea of a drive that is innate, inflexible and unwavering. I hope that, after reading this book, you now see this differently and understand that, due to the nature of desire, it will ebb and flow as your life and relationship unfolds, as having this belief is in itself good for your sex life.

This normal ebb and flow is where sexual currency can be so vital. Relating to each other as sexual people not only meets some of the motivations each of you might have for sex (feeling attractive, feeling connected), but allows you to maintain a sexual connection no matter what else is going on for you or however 'time poor' you are. A good example of this is the experience of becoming parents for the first time. We know from research that almost 90% of new parents report at least one concern about sex in the first year after having a baby,[10] and in Chapter 6 I mentioned that sexual satisfaction can be at its lowest during a couple's lifetime in the first few years of having small children. Being new parents creates obvious challenges for sex in all the ways we have spoken about (tiredness, increased household tasks, changes in body image, less time together as a couple, stress, increased distraction, etc.), but also in the biological ways we mentioned (especially tiredness). Having young children, therefore, is a time when many couples can expect there to be multiple barriers to their pre-existing sex life, in a way that might require both an acceptance that this is usual and nothing to worry about, but also that they should find ways to maintain sexual connection in the absence (or reduction) of sex.

Importantly, creating a culture of sexual currency even outside of having an active 'sex life' (by that I mean partaking in sexual acts together) maintains that scaffold which allows an easier climb to sexual activity when the moment is right. Not maintaining a culture of sexual currency, or of sexual connection, in times of low sexual activity not only means there's a risk that some of the needs that sex serves are not met, but it can leave couples with a sense that restarting sex again feels awkward or jolting. When I see couples like this for sex therapy, they often describe their relationship in terms of it feeling non-sexual (like 'brother and sister'; or 'sister and sister', if a female couple). What they mean by this is 'we've not related to each other sexually for so long that it's started to feel odd to even contemplate that'. It's this dynamic that maintaining sexual currency avoids.

Being new parents isn't the only life stage or transition during which a couple can benefit from considering the role that increasing sexual currency can have on maintaining a good sexual connection. Any situation which puts the time or inclination to keep sex a priority in jeopardy fits. This might be around work stress, moving house, feeling time pressured around family demands, through ill health, the menopause or when caring for someone else. The mistake couples often make is perceiving that it is the act of sex itself that matters, the physical release – even more: penetrative sex. But as we spoke about in Chapter 5, it is rarely the act of sex itself that motivates us to move towards sex with someone else but rather the need that it is meeting. These needs, if you remember, might be about closeness, excitement, intimacy, feeling wanted, resolving conflict, expressing attraction or 'feeling alive', for example. In a period of lower sexual interaction for whatever reason, understanding and nurturing these needs in other ways can help relationships survive when sex is off the menu. Let's look at Anna and Doug, whose experience of a significant life event affected their sex life.

Anna and Doug had been together fifteen years when they came to see me due to differences in desire, which was causing problems in their relationship. Anna had been feeling like having sex less in the last few years, partly, she thought, as she was experiencing early menopausal symptoms and had noticed a change in her mood and sleep, which was making her not feel like herself. Partly it was because she was caring for her sister, who had recently received a diagnosis of cancer. Anna felt like sex was the last thing she wanted to be thinking about and was feeling less receptive to sex with Doug. This was showing itself in reduced sexual stimuli between them, sometimes because she experienced Doug's pleas for sex as irritating and she wanted to avoid them. Once we got talking, it transpired that Anna perceived Doug's repeated requests for sex, or 'jokes' about how long it had been, as insensitive and hurtful. After all, she knew that men could be 'sex mad', but she experienced this as frivolous and disrespectful when there was so much more going on.

Anna was making assumptions about Doug's motivations for sex based on societal views of male desire (i.e. 'men always want sex', 'men have a need for physical release') and interpreting this as unimportant and insensitive. During the course of therapy we spent some time understanding their motivations for sex and the function that sex served in the relationship. We learned that Doug was actually motivated to have sex when he wanted to feel close to Anna, and that, over the course of her sister's diagnosis and illness, he had become increasingly worried about Anna's mortality and preoccupied with her becoming ill. He was craving closeness with Anna more than ever, at a time where she was restricting her affection for him, for fear of turning him on or 'giving him the wrong idea'. Anna was shocked to hear about how Doug really felt, and understanding what sex meant for him totally changed her feelings towards him when he expressed how he missed it or when he suggested it. Doug reassured Anna that being physically intimate together – whether it was sex or not – would make him feel better, and Anna was really happy to bring this back, given her new knowledge. Anna and Doug found that Anna's new understanding of Doug's motivations, changing her entrenched beliefs from 'he just wants to satisfy a physical urge' to 'he adores me and is also frightened for the future', reignited their sexual relationship, as sex took on an important and life-affirming meaning in a time of heightened mortality and stress.

The lesson from all of this for couples wanting to maintain a good sex life, despite the challenges that will undoubtedly come their way, is to understand exactly what is missing when 'sex' is and to find other ways to meet these needs until things return to an even keel.

How to deal with changing needs

Our sexuality doesn't remain static over the course of our life-time. Our sexual confidence, likes, dislikes, preferences, what we find erotic, our bodily function and ability to experience physical sensations are constantly changing. As a society we would do well to hold this in mind more when thinking about sex over the course of our sexually active years on the planet. It is certainly the case that some people's sexual problems at any life stage are a direct con-sequence of their sexual relationship not being able to adapt to these changes successfully, not the changes themselves.

The assumption of sex and sexuality as static can discourage us from having useful conversations about where we might like our sex lives to go, what changes we might like in how we do things or how changes in our identity might be indicative of new possibilities for sex. For example, women generally report fewer concerns about body image the longer they have been with a partner.[11] Women also report higher levels of sexual assertion, and therefore sexual satisfaction, as they age.[12] For some women, this can show itself in a new-found sexual confidence and feeling of wanting more variety of sexual expression as they move through life. The myth of women reaching their 'sexual peak' at an older age to men is not about sexual function per se but an awareness that (sadly) it can take women decades to shake off the restraints of body-image oppression, lack of knowledge about their genitals, acceptance of the orgasm gap and restrictions on assertiveness in order to be able to know about and demand the types of sex that they need. This increase in sexual confidence and satisfaction is to be celebrated, but the relationship women find themselves in needs to be able not just to withstand this change but adapt to it.

It's normal to develop new preferences in sexual touch, want to try out new things or suddenly develop a new interest and want to try out something different. The danger comes when we develop a relationship culture which does not support this, either because the way in which we have defined sex has become predictable and fixed, so there's no room for change, or the part we've got used to playing sexually has become predictable, or because we have not nurtured a concept of sex as flexible and ever changing, and so suggesting a change feels too 'out of the blue' or a big deal.

One of the ways I often talk about couples creating this culture of anticipated change and growth in their sexual relationships is to create a ritual of regular review and conversation about sex which follows three key lines of enquiry:

- What's been going well in our sex life that we want to continue?

- What would we like to do more of in our sex life and how can we pre-empt barriers that might get in the way?

- What new directions might we want to explore in our sex life? What would we like to try out together or alone, or learn more about?

It's useful to get into the habit of having this type of conversation regularly, linked to another date or event, for example, as part of a New Year's Day 'looking forward' conversation, linked to an anniversary, or as a ritual on a yearly summer's holiday. Building in this kind of checking-in and future-focused conversation about sex circumvents the need to only talk about sex when there is a problem, which is often the hardest time to respond and react to feedback. It is also likely to mean that conversations about sex become more positive as, by the nature of this type of discussion, sexual problems are more likely to have been avoided by pre-emptive conversations about building in changing needs and wants around sex.

Apart from changing preferences, tastes and sexual identity, there are also physical changes happening throughout the course of our lives. We often think of changes in bodily function, health and ability as negatives for sexual function, but they don't need to be.

In fact, forced modifications to our sex lives as a result of physical changes can be a time of golden opportunity in so many ways. They provide an opportunity to break free of predictable, societally dictated sexual scripts and habits or the routines we can easily fall into with the same person over time. These changes can allow us the opportunity to experience new sensations, new ways of being, or to bring different definitions to what sex means. These aspects of life challenges don't get the airtime they should, in my opinion, in terms of the potential impact they could have on revitalizing sexual expression and satisfaction.

Consider pregnancy, for example. Pregnancy is a time of intense physical, psychological and relational transition. It is also a time of well-documented changes in sexual function. Desire might increase or decrease, penetrative sex might feel more or less welcome, orgasms might change in their trigger, intensity or sensation. These experiences can provide great opportunities for novel experiences of pleasure, expression and desire if we welcome them. It we don't, they might show themselves in sexual problems (which are actually very common in pregnancy). Adapting to new sexual positions that don't put pressure on the abdomen from the second trimester onwards can be challenging for couples who only ever have sex in the 'missionary' position. Equally, adapting to a sudden dislike of penetrative sex can be difficult if you have reduced your sex life to very little else. For some people, however, experimentation in pregnancy can lead to the emergence of new sexual preferences that would otherwise have gone undiscovered. Having to communicate and adapt in times of physical change opens doors around sex that might have otherwise stayed closed. The benefits of this adaptation is also true for the impact of ageing and health-related sexual changes, such as age-related declines in genital sensitivity, difficulties with erectile function linked to ill health or changes in mobility. As with many other aspects of our sex life, it is the way we respond to these challenges, not the challenges themselves, that dictates our future sexual satisfaction.

It's important to note that, for some women, going through the menopause can have a negative impact on desire, and this is a good example of how our sex life might need to temporarily or permanently adapt to our changing needs. The physical and psychological impact of the menopause – hot flushes, sleep difficulties, vaginal dryness, painful sex and low mood – are well documented, and for obvious reasons (which by this stage in the book you will be super familiar with) reduce desire. Who wants someone touching them when they feel as though they are in an oven and dripping with sweat? Who wants to continue a sex life with their partner if it's only been penetrative vaginal sex for the last fifteen years and penetrative sex now hurts? One piece of good news about this is that this doesn't happen for everyone, and for many women not having to think about contraception or periods brings with it a new sense of sexual freedom. The other good news is that research suggests that how your sex life was pre-menopause and your feelings towards your partner are more reliable predictors of how your sex life will be post-menopause than your oestrogen levels.[13] This makes sense when you think about it, as hormones are essential to the process of arousal and desire but, as desire is a largely a psychological, relational and social event, these other aspects are key to how easily desire can emerge. When you add in the other life changes which might be happening for women around the same time, such as the possibility of having elderly parents to look after, experiencing being seen as 'less sexual' by society, being in a long-term relationship, and the increased chance of a partner of a roughly similar age having a sexual problem, we can see how these things might also contribute. The menopause is certainly a time of physical change for women which can bring with it transitions in sex and desire, but it is important to remember that there are effective physical treatments for these symptoms, such as hormone replacement therapy (HRT), local oestrogens and the use of vaginal moisturizers and lubes which can really help to alleviate symptoms. Research tells us that many people in mid-life and older don't feel comfortable talking to their doctor or health-care provider about their sex life.[14] This is unfortunate, and a byproduct of the impact of ageist (and inaccurate) ideas of people in mid-life and beyond being less sexual, as well as the challenge of a lifetime of being socialised not to talk about sex. Please do talk to your health-care provider if you are experiencing symptoms which are affecting your life in this way, so that you can be supported effectively during this transition.

Is sex a priority?

For some people, sex is the most important, or one of the most important, things in a relationships; for others not so much. It's possible that you are reading this book because you are somebody who rates sex as important, and doing so is one of the ways in which you are treating it as such. It's also possible that you are reading this book because society *tells you* that sex is important, but actually, for you, it's not so much of a big deal. Whichever way you look at it, there's no doubt that, for many couples, the research shows that sexual satisfaction is good for relationship satisfaction, even if it's not the most important thing.

I firmly believe that, if we feel sex is important, we should treat it as such, by taking purposeful and intentional action to prioritize it. I also feel that the way in which sex and desire are framed to us in society is that 'it shouldn't need work' and 'it should just happen', which totally gets in the way of us knowing how to action prioritizing it. You don't stay healthy without taking purposeful and intentional action around your diet and exercise, and sex is similar, except possibly more challenging, as it involves the understanding, communication and commitment to action of someone else. A change in mindset, therefore, is what's needed to understand what needs to be done and to choose to do it.

We lead busy lives, but we are constantly making choices about how to spend our time and we need to consider the impact that this will have on our lives and relationships. The problem with how we've perhaps seen sex until now is that we haven't thought of it as something we need to dedicate time to. Perhaps now we have identified the multitude of reasons and ways in which we might give it more priority, we might have to consider other sacrifices or changes in our routine to make this possible. After all, I'm not sure there are many of us who routinely sit twiddling our thumbs and have time to spare. These decisions about prioritizing are tough, but there is often room for some compromise. For example, it can be hard to make time for self-expanding activities as a couple, especially if you have young children and can't afford a babysitter. But it might be that you make a commitment to doing this once a month. If this isn't possible, there is no reason you can't swap one night of TV viewing a week for a night dedicated to novel fun together, or other types of connection, at home. Buy some paints and try to paint each other's portrait, try to cook a complex recipe together, play a board game, plan a future project, talk about your hopes and dreams. Other useful changes, such as increasing sexual currency, don't have to take any extra time in a person's day but do require intentional effort and consideration. Creating moments of increased emotional intimacy or physical triggers for desire, such as dedicating one night a week to go to bed early after dinner and lie naked to talk – really talk – and listen will require a decision to reprioritize this over spending time with friends, scrolling through Instagram, going to the gym or whatever else.

It is, of course, your call. But I'd like you to consider that *not* taking action to prioritize sex *is* taking action, just in a different way. Your sex life is happening and unfolding on its own trajectory; the question for you is how much you want to steer it versus see in which direction it drifts.

Conclusion

I hope that, in reading this book, you have learned that female sexuality, satisfaction and desire have historically been presented to us in a way that disadvantages women's sex lives from flourishing and that the problem with 'low desire' does not lie within the bodies or minds of individual women. What I hope you are taking away is that much of this unhelpful discourse around women's sexuality is situated within our societies and gender politics (including how these biases have influenced science) and that the real truth of women's desire can set us free. By now, I hope you have understood that women's desire, albeit a complex response to a collection of factors which might require some purposeful action to be triggered, is much more than meets the eye, and is very closely related to our social, political, cultural and relationship circumstances than is often presented to us in soundbites in the press. Women's desire is not broken; it just needs to be understood.

I also hope you have taken away the fact that women's experience of sex, from early learning about bodily autonomy, safety and pleasure, is heavily influenced by gender politics around whose needs or pleasure is privileged. Similarly, societal messages about women's sexuality and sex more generally, plus the objectification of women's bodies, can disadvantage desire in a way that we are not always consciously aware of, but we *do* have the power to take action around. This can be a personal movement, such as in how we decide to relate to sex or our bodies through what we choose to expose ourselves to in magazines/social media, or by participating in wider social movements grounded in feminism, such as #MeToo. I hope you feel angry about the forces that impact on women's sexuality, not just so you can more easily reject some of the less helpful forces in your own sex life but so you have the inclination to be part of facilitating change for younger generations to come.

I hope that this book has taken you on a journey of understanding how you relate to sex and what you need from it in a way that is reassuring for your sex life, regardless of whether a good sex life for you is letting go of the importance of sex, or on focusing more attention on it. My aim is to give you the knowledge and skills to futureproof your sex life, and I hope that, no matter how good or in crisis your sex life feels at the moment, you have learned things that will not only make you feel empowered to make it better right now, but also arm you with the information and science you need to create a lifetime of good sex, no matter what life throws at you.

After all, the key to sexual satisfaction and desire over the course of your life is to understand it and then make a decision to move towards what will help, based on these new understandings. This is how our sex lives can continue to improve over time rather than stagnate or decline. I hope that this book has given you new understandings and ideas of how you can do this for yourself. The rest is up to you.

Here's to your revolution.

Acknowledgements

I would like to acknowledge and sincerely thank the following people, whom, without their faith, support and encouragement this book would not have been possible.

Firstly, my wonderful editor Anna Steadman, of Headline Home, for providing the guidance, support and expertise for me to put my thoughts and words into *Mind The Gap*. I have total respect and admiration for you and wish to thank you for having so much faith in my initial vision for this book and in my writing from the outset.

Huge thanks also to my agent Julia Silk, of Kingsford Campbell, for helping me navigate the literary world, creating this opportunity and for the support, encouragement and phone calls along the way. I'm so glad our paths crossed!

Thanks to the rest of the incredible team at Headline Home, particularly my publicist Jessica Farrugia, Caroline Young for creating such a bold, modern cover but also for listening to my preferences throughout the process and Anna Hervé for her fantastic attention to detail and thoughtfulness in refining this book at the copy-edit stage.

Without the contribution of sex scientists and researchers all over the world, too numerous to mention, this book would have been purely clinical opinion, and I wish to thank them for the work that they do in helping all of us understand sexuality better. I have learned (and am still learning) every day from the work that you do. I would particularly like to thank Professor Lori Brotto, Professor Cynthia Graham, Professor Helen King and Professor Kirstin Mitchell for their comments on early versions of this manuscript, and also for their professional guidance, inspiration and friendship. Lori and Cindy, I have not forgotten that lovely meal we had on the Titanic(!) and how humble and generous you both were (and still are) about the things that you have achieved and in your support.

I also wish to thank all of the women who have attended my online desire workshops and the women and couples that I have worked with in sex therapy over the last few decades who have taught me so much about working with sex. It's always a privilege to sit in a room with clients and I am grateful for that every day. I am moved, enthused, excited, invigorated and thankful that you allow me to share in your journey to a better sexual life and seeing the impact of this on you and your relationships has been a motivation to me to convey some of these ideas on a wider level.

Thank you to all my friends who have read chapters, provided encouragement, support and a listening ear during this process. Particular thanks to Paul Lawrenson, Steven Thwaite, Chloe Potter, Lindy Fittall, Kate Baxter, Tamzin Davis, Lizzie Thorne, and Jyothi Parekh who have all heard more about this book than they needed to over many meals out and whose enthusiasm for it has been a huge source of motivation along the way.

Thank you to fellow authors and friends Maisie Hill, Sarah Hyndman and David Bodanis for being a source of encouragement, inspiration and for being the 'yes, do it!' cheerleading team when I was offered this opportunity. It was so useful to have your experience and perspective on the book writing process. Thank you to all of my Paragon family for being a constant source of friendship and inspiration, and for listening to me talk about the book when I'm supposed to be training, particularly Jessica Shivji and Rob Taliesin Owen. Thanks also to Rae Langford for her friendship, enthusiasm and support and for providing a tranquil space to write when I needed it.

Thank you to the rest of the Havelock Clinic team, Dr Ali Mears, Dr Jane Ashby, Dr Michael Yates, Sarah Wolujewicz and Katy Harrad for teaching me so much, being such inspirations and allowing me to take my foot off the accelerator for a few months to focus on this book. I'm so proud to work with the best in the business and I am forever grateful for having you as my colleagues. Thank you also to all of the incredible team at 56 Dean Street who have provided encouragement and flexibility over the last few months. It really is a joy to work with you.

Thank you to the psychology teacher and my first supervisor who told me to give up on my dreams of being a clinical psychologist as it was 'too competitive' and I was not 'academic enough'. I'm glad I was too young and enthusiastic back then to listen to you. Real thanks and appreciation to Glenda Fredman, who taught me the joy of systemic therapy and how to truly work well with couples. I hope you see the influence of the seed you planted within me in this book. Thank you for being such an inspiration to me professionally. I use your teachings in every therapy session I do.

Lastly, I could not have succeeded in this endeavour without the support of my family, who have sacrificed and given themselves in a way that they always do to support me in my goals. Thank you to my mum, dad, brother and sister-in-law Anna for unconditional love and bearing with my lack of visits up north, the endless childcare and me needing to work all the time. Thank you to my two boys for being magnificent and accepting that I've worked a lot recently – I can play now, boys! Get the Lego out!

My final and most important thanks to my partner AJ, for whom this book is dedicated, and for whom I am grateful for every single day. Thank you for the online shops, the washing, for taking the kids swimming, for talking me out of my doubts, for the (very slow) reading, and most importantly for your unfaltering belief in me and this book. I adore you.

Notes

1. A brief history of sex, science and gender politics

1. E.g.: https://quod.lib.umich.edu/w/wsfh/0642292.0033.009/--marriage-calculations-in-the-eighteenth-century?rgn=main; view=fulltext.
2. Dabhoiwala, F., *The Origins of Sex: A History of the First Sexual Revolution* (London: Allen Lane, 2012).
3. Forde, K., Beddard, H. and Angel, K., *The Institute of Sexology* (London: Wellcome Collection/Prestel Publishing, 2014).
4. *Diagnostic and Statistical Manual of Mental Disorders*, 3rd ed. (Washington, DC: American Psychiatric Association, 1980).
5. Ellis, H., *Sexual Inversion* (1896); republished in *Studies in the Psychology of Sex*, vol. 2, 'Sexual Inversion' (CreateSpace Independent Publishing Platform, 2014).
6. Kaplan, H.S., 'Hypoactive Sexual Desire', *Journal of Sex & Marital Therapy*, 3:3–9 (1979).
7. Jaspers, L., Feys, F., Bramer, W.M., Franco, O.H., Leusink, P. and Laan, E.M., 'Efficacy and Safety of Flibanserin for the Treatment of Hypoactive Sexual Desire Disorder in Women: A Systematic Review and Meta-Analysis', *JAMA Internal Medicine*, 176, 453–62 (2016).

8. Working Group for a New View of Women's Sexual Problems (2000): *The New View Manifesto: A New View of Women's Sexual Problems*, http://www.fsd-alert.org/manifesto5.asp. Accessed 28 February 2019: Kaschak, E. and Tiefer, L. (eds.), *A New View of Womens' Sexual Problems* (New York, NY: Haworth Press, 2001).

9. *Diagnostic and Statistical Manual of Mental Disorders*, 5th ed. (Washington, DC: American Psychiatric Association, 2013).

2. Mind the gap – statistics around sex and desire

1. See all key findings and papers at http://www.natsal.ac.uk/home.aspx.

2. Wellings, K., Palmer, M.J., Machiyama K. and Slaymaker, E., 'Changes in, and Factors Associated with, Frequency of Sex in Britain: Evidence from Three National Surveys of Sexual Attitudes and Lifestyles (Natsal)', *British Medical Journal*, 365:1525 (2019).

3. Mitchell, K.R., Mercer, C.H., Ploubidis, G.B., et al., 'Sexual Function in Britain: Findings from the Third National Survey of Sexual Attitudes and Lifestyles', *The Lancet*, 382 (2013).

4. Mitchell, Kirstin R., Jones, Kyle G., Wellings, Kaye, Johnson, Anne M., Graham, Cynthia A., Datta, Jessica, Copas, Andrew J., Bancroft, John, Sonnenberg, Pam, Macdowall, Wendy, Field, Nigel, and Mercer, Catherine H., 'Estimating the Prevalence of Sexual Function Problems: The Impact of Morbidity Criteria', *Journal of Sex Research* (2015).

5. Taylor, P., Funk, C. and Clark, A., 'Generation Gap in Values, Behaviors: As Marriage and Parenthood Drift Apart, Public is Concerned about Social Impact', Pew Research Centre (2007).

6. Burleson, M.H., Trevathan, W.R. and Todd, M., 'In the Mood for Love or Vice Versa? Exploring the Relations among Sexual Activity, Physical Affection, Affect, and Stress in the Daily Lives

of Mid-Aged Women', *Archives of Sexual Behavior*, 36, 357–68 (2007).

7. Muise, A., Impett, E.A., Desmarais, S. and Kogan, A., 'Keeping the Spark Alive: Being Motivated to Meet a Partner's Sexual Needs Sustains Sexual Desire in Long-Term Romantic Relationships', *Social Psychological and Personality Sciences*, 4, 267–73 (2013).

8. Fallis, E.E., Rehman, U.S., Woody, E.Z. and Purdon, C., 'The Longitudinal Association of Relationship Satisfaction and Sexual Satisfaction in Long-Term Relationships', *Journal of Family Psychology*, 30, 822–31 (2016).

9. Mitchell, K.R., Mercer, C.H., Ploubidis, G.B., et al., 'Sexual Function in Britain: Findings from the Third National Survey of Sexual Attitudes and Lifestyles', *The Lancet*, 382 (2013).

10. Sprecher S., 'Sexual Satisfaction in Premarital Relationships: Associations with Satisfaction, Love, Commitment, and Stability', *Journal of Sex Research*, 39:190–96 (2002); Heiman, J.R., Long, J.S., Smith, S.N., Fisher, W.A., Sand, M.S. and Rosen, R.C., 'Sexual Satisfaction and Relationship Happiness in Midlife and Older Couples in Five Countries', *Archives of Sexual Behavior*, 40, 741–53 (2011).

11. Brezsnyak, M. and Whisman, M.A., 'Sexual Desire and Relationship Functioning: The Effects of Marital Satisfaction and Power', *Journal of Sex and Marital Therapy*, 30, 199–217 (2004); Hinchliff, S. and Gott, M., 'Intimacy, Commitment, and Adaptation: Sexual Relationships within Long-Term Marriages', *Journal of Social and Personal Relationships*, 21, 595–609 (2004).

12. Regan, P.C., 'The Role of Sexual Desire and Sexual Activity in Dating Relationships', *Social Behavior and Personality*, 28, 51–9 (2000).

13. Traeen, B., 'When Sex becomes a Duty', *Sexual and Relationship Therapy*, 23(1), 61–84 (2008).

14. Revicki, D.A., Fisher, W., Rosen, R.C., Kuppermann, M., Margolis, M.K. and Hanes, V., 'The Impact of Hypoactive Sexual Desire Disorder (HSDD) on Women and Their Relationships: Qualitative Data from Patient Focus Groups', *Journal of Sexual Medicine*, 7(3), 124–125 (2010).

15. Muise, A. and Impett, E.A., 'Applying Theories of Communal Motivation to Sexuality. Social and Personality Psychology', 455–67 (2016).

16. Mitchell, K.R., King, M., Nazareth, I. and Wellings, K., 'Managing Sexual Difficulties: A Qualitative Investigation of Coping Strategies', *Journal of Sex Research*, 48:4, 325–33 (2011).

17. Klusmann, D., 'Sexual Motivation and the Duration of Partnership', *Archives of Sexual Behavior*, 31, 275–87 (2002); Sims, K.E. and Meana, M., 'Why Did Passion Wane? A Qualitative Study of Married Women's Attributions for Declines in Sexual Desire', *Journal of Sex and Marital Therapy*, 36(4), 360–80 (2010).

18. Velten, J. and Margraf, J., 'Satisfaction Guaranteed? How Actor, Partner, and Relationship Factors Impact Sexual Satisfaction within Partnerships', *PLoS ONE*, 12, e0172855 (2017); Acevedo, B.P. and Aron, A., 'Does a Long-Term Relationship Kill Romantic Love?', *Review of General Psychology*, 13(1), 59–65 (2009).

19. Both, S., Everaerd, W., Laan, E. and Janssen, E., 'Desire Emerges from Excitement: A Psychophysiological Perspective on Sexual Motivation', in Janssen, E. (ed.), *The Psychophysiology of Sex* (Bloomington, IN: Indiana University Press, 2007), pp. 327–39.

20. Murray, S. and Milhausen, R., 'Factors Impacting Women's Sexual Desire: Examining Long-Term Relationships in Emerging Adulthood', *Canadian Journal of Human Sexuality*, 21, 101–15 (2012).

21. Herbenick, D., Mullinax, M. and Mark, K., 'Sexual Desire Discrepancy as a Feature, Not a Bug, of Long-Term

Relationships: Women's Self-Reported Strategies for Modulating
Sexual Desire', *Journal of Sexual Medicine*, 11, 2196–206 (2014).

22. Dawson, S.J. and Chivers, M.L., 'Gender Differences and
Similarities in Sexual Desire', *Current Sexual Health Reports*,
6:211–19 (2014).

23. Basson, R., Brotto, L.A., Petkau, J.A. and Labrie, F., 'Role of
Androgens in Women's Sexual Dysfunction', *Menopause: The
Journal of the North American Menopause Society*, 17(5), 962–71
2010).

24. Hyde, J.S., Bigler, R.S., Joel, D., Tate, C.C. and van Anders, S.M.,
'The Future of Sex and Gender in Psychology: Five Challenges
to the Gender Binary', *American Psychologist*. Advance online
publication (2018).

25. Murray, S. and Milhausen, R., 'Sexual Desire and Relationship
Duration in Young Men and Women', *Journal of Sex & Marital
Therapy*, 38, 28 (2012).

26. Martin, Wednesday, *Untrue: Why Nearly Everything We Believe
about Women and Lust and Infidelity is Untrue* (London: Scribe
Publications, 2018).

27. Laumann, E.O., Nicolosi, A., Glasser, D.B., Paik, A., Gingell, C.,
Moreira, E., et al., 'Sexual Problems among Women and Men
Aged 40–80 Years: Prevalence and Correlates Identified in the
Global Study of Sexual Attitudes and Behaviors', *International
Journal of Impotence Research*, 17, 39–57 (2005).

28. Cawood, E.H. and Bancroft, J., 'Steroid Hormones, the
Menopause, Sexuality and Wellbeing of Women', *Psychological
Medicine*, 26, 925–36 (1996); Cain, V.S., Johannes, C.B., Avis,
N.E., Mohr, B., Schocken, M., Skurnick, J. and Ory, M., 'Sexual
Functioning and Practices in a Multi-Ethnic Study of Midlife
Women: Baseline Results from SWAN', *Journal of Sex Research*,
40:3, 266–76 (2003); Avis, N.E., Zhao, X., Johannes, C.B., Ory,
M., Brockwell, S. and Greendale, G.A., 'Correlates of Sexual
Function among Multi-Ethnic Middle-Aged Women: Results

from the Study of Women's Health across the Nation (SWAN)', *Menopause*, 12, 385–98 (2005).

29. Chivers, M.L. and Brotto, L.A., 'Controversies of Women's Sexual Arousal and Desire', *European Psychologist*, 22(1), 5–26 (2017).

3. Gaps in the foundations

1. Palmer, M.J., Clarke, L., Ploubidis, G.B., Mercer, C.H., Gibson, L.J., Johnson, A.M., Copas, A.J. and Wellings, K., 'Is "Sexual Competence" at First Heterosexual Intercourse Associated with Subsequent Sexual Health Status?', *Journal of Sex Research*, 54:1, 91–104 (2017).
2. Wellings, K., Nanchahal, K., Macdowall, W., McManus, S., Erens, B., Mercer, C.H. and Field, J., 'Sexual Behaviour in Britain: Early Heterosexual Experience', *The Lancet*, 358(9296), 1843–50 (2001).
3. Blechner, M.J., 'The Clitoris: Anatomical and Psychological Issues, Studies in Gender and Sexuality', 18:3, 190–200 (2017).
4. O'Connell, H., Sanjeevan, K. and Hutson, J., 'Anatomy of the Clitoris', *Journal of Urology*: 174, 1189–95 (2005).
5. Carvalheira, A., and Leal, I., 'Masturbation among Women: Associated Factors and Sexual Response in a Portuguese Community Sample', *Journal of Sex & Marital Therapy*, 39(4), 347–67 (2013).
6. Brewer, G. and Hendrie, C.A., 'Evidence to Suggest that Copulatory Vocalizations in Women are Not a Reflexive Consequence of Orgasm', *Archives of Sexual Behavior*: 40(3), 559–64 (2011); Hite, S., *The Hite Report: A Nationwide Study of Female Sexuality* (Dell Publishing Co.,1976); Kinsey, A.C., Pomeroy, W.B., Martin, C.E. and Gebhard, P.H., 'Sexual Behavior in the Human Female', Saunders (1953).

7. Frederick, D.A., St John, H.K., Garcia, J.R. and Lloyd, E.A., 'Differences in Orgasm Frequency among Gay, Lesbian, Bisexual, and Heterosexual Men and Women in a US National Sample', *Archives Sexual Behaviour*, 47:273–88 (2018).
8. Armstrong, E.A., England, P. and Fogarty, A.C.K., 'Accounting for Women's Orgasm and Sexual Enjoyment in College Hookups and Relationships', *American Sociological Review*, 77(3) 435–62 (2012).
9. http://www.tandfonline.com/doi/abs/10.1080/00224499.2017.1303437?journalCode=hjsr20.
10. Fugl-Meyer, K.S., Oberg, K., Lundberg, P.O., Lewin, B. and Fugl-Meyer, A., 'On Orgasm, Sexual Techniques, and Erotic Perceptions in 18- to 74-year-old Swedish Women', *Journal of Sexual Medicine*, 3, 56 (2006).
11. Purnine, D.M., Carey, M.P. and Jorgensen, R.S. 'Gender Differences Regarding Preferences for Specific Heterosexual Practices', *Journal of Sex & Marital Therapy*, 20(4), 271–87 (1994).
12. Blair, K.L., Cappell, J. and Pukall, C.F., 'Not All Orgasms were Created Equal: Differences in Frequency and Satisfaction of Orgasm Experiences by Sexual Activity in Same-Sex versus Mixed-Sex Relationships', *Journal of Sex Research*, 55:6, 719–33 (2018).
13. Frederick, D.A., St John, H.K., Garcia, J.R. and Lloyd, E.A., 'Differences in Orgasm Frequency among Gay, Lesbian, Bisexual, and Heterosexual Men and Women in a US National Sample', *Archives Sexual Behaviour*, 47:273–88 (2018).
14. Bell, S.N. and McClelland, S.I., 'When, If, and How: Young Women Contend with Orgasmic Absence', *Journal of Sex Research*, 55:6, 679–91 (2018).
15. Wade, L. D., Kremer, E. C. and Brown, J. 'The Incidental Orgasm: The Presence of Clitoral Knowledge and the Absence of Orgasm for Women', *Women and Health*, 42, 117–38.

16. Summarized in Frederick, D.A., St John, H.K., Garcia, J.R. and Lloyd, E.A., 'Differences in Orgasm Frequency among Gay, Lesbian, Bisexual, and Heterosexual Men and Women in a US National Sample', *Archives Sexual Behaviour*, 47:273–88 (2018).

17. Lloyd, E., *The Case for Female Orgasm: Bias in the Science of Evolution* (Cambridge, MA: Harvard University Press, 2005).

18. Kleinplatz, P.J. and Menard, A.D., 'Building Blocks towards Optimal Sexuality: Constructing a Conceptual Model', *Family Journal: Counselling and Therapy for Couples and Families*, vol. 15, 1, 72–8 (2007).

4. Sex in our society

1. E.g.: see https://www.telegraph.co.uk/women/life/happened-primary-school-went-gender-neutral/.

2. Gagnon, J. and Simon, W., 'Sexual Conduct: The Social Origins of Human Sexuality', Aldine (1973).

3. Alarie, M., 'Sleeping with Younger Men: Women's Accounts of Sexual Interplay in Age-Hypogamous Intimate Relationships', *Journal of Sex Research* (2019); Blair, K.L., Cappell, J. and Pukall, C.F., 'Not All Orgasms were Created Equal: Differences in Frequency and Satisfaction of Orgasm Experiences by Sexual Activity in Same-Sex versus Mixed-Sex Relationships', *Journal of Sex Research*, 55:6, 719–73 (2018); Séguin, L.J. and Milhausen, R.R., 'Not All Fakes are Created Equal: Examining the Relationships between Men's Motives for Pretending Orgasm and Levels of Sexual Desire, and Relationship and Sexual Satisfaction', *Sexual and Relationship Therapy*, 31:2, 159–75 (2016); Gewirtz-Meydan, A. and Ayalon, L., 'Why Do Older Adults Have Sex? Approach and Avoidance Sexual Motives among Older Women and Men', *Journal of Sex Research* (2018); Klein, V., Imhoff, R., Reininger, K.M. and Briken, P., 'Perceptions of

Sexual Script Deviation in Women and Men, *Archives of Sexual Behavior*, 48:631–44 (2019); Chadwick, S.B. and van Anders, S.M., 'Do Women's Orgasms Function as a Masculinity Achievement for Men?', *Journal of Sex Research*, 54, 1141–1152 (2017).

4. Blair, K.L., Cappell, J. and Pukall, C.F., 'Not All Orgasms were Created Equal: Differences in Frequency and Satisfaction of Orgasm Experiences by Sexual Activity in Same-Sex versus Mixed-Sex Relationships', *Journal of Sex Research*, 55:6, 719–73 (2018); Holmberg, D. and Blair, K.L., 'Sexual Desire, Communication, Satisfaction, and Preferences of Men and Women in Same-Sex versus Mixed-Sex Relationships', *Journal of Sex Research*, 46(1):57–66 (2009).

5. Rosenkrantz, D.E. and Mark, K.P., 'The Sociocultural Context of Sexually Diverse Women's Sexual Desire', *Sexuality and Culture*, 22: 220 (2018).

6. https://www.ofcom.org.uk/__data/assets/pdf_file/0021/149124/adults-media-use-and-attitudes-report.pdf.

7. The Erika Lust not-for-profit site, www.thepornconversation.org, reports that a third of internet traffic is porn.

8. Mercer, C.H., Tanton, C., Prah, P. et al., 'Changes in Sexual Attitudes and Lifestyles in Britain through the Life Course and over Time: Findings from the National Surveys of Sexual Attitudes and Lifestyles (Natsal)', *The Lancet* (published online 26 November 2013).

9. Séguin, L.J., Rodrigue, C. and Lavigne, J., 'Consuming Ecstasy: Representations of Male and Female Orgasm in Mainstream Pornography', *Journal of Sex Research*, 55:3, 348356 (2018).

10. Hurlbert, D.F., 'The Role of Assertiveness in Female Sexuality: A Comparative Study between Sexually Assertive and Sexually Non-Assertive Women', *Journal of Sex & Marital Therapy*, 17, 183–90 (1991).

11. Muehlenhard, C.L. and Shippee, S.K., 'Men's and Women's

Reports of Pretending Orgasm', *Journal of Sex Research*, 47:6, 55–567 (2010).

12. Shirazi, T., Renfro, K.J., Lloyd, E. and Wallen, K., 'Women's Experience of Orgasm during Intercourse: Question Semantics Affect Women's Reports and Men's Estimates of Orgasm Occurrence', *Archives Sexual Behaviour*, 47:605–13 (2018).

13. Lewis, R. and Marston, C., 'Oral Sex, Young People, and Gendered Narratives of Reciprocity', *Journal of Sex Research*, 53:7, 776–787 (2016).

14. Graham, C.A., Sanders, S.A., Milhausen, R.R. and McBride, K.R. 'Turning On and Turning Off: A Focus Group Study of the Factors that Affect Women's Sexual Arousal', *Archives of Sexual Behavior*, 33, 527–38 (2004).

15. Davison, T.E. and McCabe, M.P., 'Relationships between Men's and Women's Body Image and Their Psychological, Social, and Sexual Functioning', *Sex Roles*, 52, 463–75 (2005).

16. Fredrickson, B.L. and Roberts, T.A., 'Objectification Theory', *Psychology of Women Quarterly*, 21, 173–206 (1997).

17. Summarized in Dosch, Alessandra, Ghisletta, Paolo, and Van der Linden, Martial, 'Body Image in Dyadic and Solitary Sexual Desire: The Role of Encoding Style and Distracting Thoughts', *Journal of Sex Research*, 53:9, 1193–206 (2016).

18. Claudat, K. and Warren, C.S., 'Self-Objectification, Body Self-Consciousness during Sexual Activities, and Sexual Satisfaction in College Women', *Body Image*, 11, 509 (2014).

19. Robbins, A.R. and Reissing, E.D., 'Out of "Objectification Limelight"? The Contribution of Body Appreciation to Sexual Adjustment in Midlife Women', *Journal of Sex Research* (2017).

20. Frederick, D.A., Lever, J., Gillespie, B.J. and Garcia, J.R., 'What Keeps Passion Alive? Sexual Satisfaction is Associated with Sexual Communication, Mood Setting, Sexual Variety, Oral Sex, Orgasm, and Sex Frequency in a National US Study',

Journal of Sex Research, 54:2, 186–20 (2017).

21. Ward, L.M., Jerald, M., Avery, L. and Cole, E.R., 'Following Their Lead? Connecting Mainstream Media Use to Black Women's Gender Beliefs and Sexual Agency', *Journal of Sex Research* (2019).

22. https://www.theguardian.com/commentisfree/2015/mar/25/women-of-color-police-sexual-assault-racist-criminal-justice.

5. Sex in our relationships

1. Martin, Wednesday, *Untrue: Why Nearly Everything We Believe about Women and Lust and Infidelity is Untrue* (London: Scribe Publications, 2018).

2. Lehmiller, J., *Tell Me What You Want: The Science of Sexual Desire and How It Can Help You Improve Your Sex Life* (London: Robinson, 2018).

3. Mallory, A.B., Stanton, A.M. and Handy, A.B. 'Couples' Sexual Communication and Dimensions of Sexual Function: A Meta-Analysis', *Journal of Sex Research* (2019).

4. Murray, S.H., Milhausen, R.R. and Sutherland, O., 'A Qualitative Comparison of Young Women's Maintained versus Decreased Sexual Desire in Longer-Term Relationships', *Women and Therapy*, 37, 319–41 (2014).

5. Bateson, G., 'Steps to an Ecology of Mind', Chandler Publications for Health Sciences (1972).

6. Gonzalez-Rivas, S.K. and Peterson, Z.D., 'Women's Sexual Initiation in Same- and Mixed-Sex Relationships: How Often and How?', *Journal of Sex Research* (2018).

7. Kim, J.J., Muise, A. and Impett, E.A., 'Not in the Mood? How Do People Reject Their Partner for Sex and How Does It Matter? Paper presented at the Canadian Sex Research Forum, Kelowna, Canada 1 September 2015, in Muise, A., Maxwell, J.A. and Impett, E.A. (2018) What Theories and Methods from

Relationship Research Can Contribute to Sex Research', *Journal of Sex Research*, 55:4–5, 540–62 (2018).

8. Meston, C.M. and Buss, D.M., 'Why Humans Have Sex', *Archives of Sexual Behavior*, 36, 477–507 (2007).

9. Impett, E.A. and Peplau, L.A., 'Sexual Compliance: Gender, Motivational, and Relationship Perspectives', *Journal of Sex Research*, 40:1, 87–100 (2003).

10. Muise, A., Impett, E.A. and Desmarais, S., 'Getting It On versus Getting It Over With: Sexual Motivation, Desire, and Satisfaction in Intimate Bonds', *Personality and Social Psychology Bulletin*, 39, 1320–32 (2013).

11. Muise, A., Impett, E.A., Kogan, A. and Desmarais, S., 'Keeping the Spark Alive: Being Motivated to Meet a Partner's Sexual Needs Sustains Sexual Desire in Long-Term Romantic Relationships', *Social Psychological and Personality Science*, 4, 267 (2013).

12. Dewitte, M., 'Different Perspectives on the Sex-Attachment Link: Towards an Emotion-Motivational Account', *Journal of Sex Research*, 49:2–3, 105–12 (2012).

13. Sims, K.E. and Meana, M., 'Why Did Passion Wane? A Qualitative Study of Married Women's Attributions for Declines in Sexual Desire', *Journal of Sex & Marital Therapy*, 36(4), 360–80 (2010).

14. Ferreira, L.C., Fraenkel, P., Narciso, I. and Novo, R., 'Is Committed Desire Intentional? A Qualitative Exploration of Sexual Desire and Differentiation of Self in Couples', *Family Process*, 54, 308–26 (2015); Ferreira, L.C., Narciso, I., Novo, R.F. and Pereira, C.R., 'Predicting Couple Satisfaction: The Role of Differentiation of Self, Sexual Desire, and Intimacy in Heterosexual Individuals', *Sexual and Relationship Therapy*, 29, 390 (2014).

15. Rubin, H. and Campbell, L., 'Day-to-Day Changes in Intimacy Predict Heightened Relationship Passion, Sexual Occurrence,

and Sexual Satisfaction: A Dyadic Diary Analysis', *Social Psychological and Personality Science*, 3, 224–31 (2012).

16. Perel, E., *Mating in Captivity: Reconciling the Erotic and the Domestic* (New York, NY: HarperCollins, 2006).

17. Muise, A., Harasymchuk, C., Day, L.C., Bacev-Giles, C., Gere, J. and Impett, E. A., 'Broadening Your Horizons: Self-Expanding Activities Promote Desire and Satisfaction in Established Romantic Relationships', *Journal of Personality and Social Psychology*, advance online publication (2018).

18. https://www.telegraph.co.uk/news/2018/08/01/decade-smartphones-now-spend-entire-day-every-week-online/.

19. Kalmbach, D.A., Arnedt, J.T., Pillai, V. and Ciesla, J.A., 'The Impact of Sleep on Female Sexual Response and Behavior: A Pilot Study', *Journal of Sexual Medicine*, 12 :1221–32 (2015).

20. Ahlborg, T., Rudeblad, K., Linnér, S. and Linton, S., 'Sensual and Sexual Marital Contentment in Parents of Small Children – A Follow-Up Study When the First Child is Four Years Old', *Journal of Sex Research*, 45:3, 295–304 (2008).

21. Maas, M.K., McDaniel, B.T., Feinberg, M.E. and Jones D.E., 'Division of Labor and Multiple Domains of Sexual Satisfaction among First-Time Parents', *Journal of Family Issues*, 39:1, 104–27 (2015).

6. Sex in our brains

1. Both, S., Everaerd, W., Laan, E. and Janssen, E., 'Desire Emerges from Excitement: A Psychophysiological Perspective on Sexual Motivation', in Janssen, E. (ed.), *The Psychophysiology of Sex* (Bloomington, IN: Indiana University Press, 2007), pp. 327–39.

2. Toates, F.M., 'An Integrative Theoretical Framework for Understanding Sexual Motivation, Arousal, and Behavior', *Journal of Sex Research*, 46:2–3, 168–93 (2009); Singer, B. and

Toates, F.M., 'Sexual Motivation', *Journal of Sex Research*, 23:4, 481–501 (1987).

3. Chivers, M.L., Seto, M.C., Lalumière, M.L., Laan, E. and Grimbos, T., 'Agreement of Self-Reported and Genital Measures of Sexual Arousal in Men and Women: A Meta-Analysis', *Archives of Sexual Behavior*, 39, 5 (2010).

4. Chivers, M.L., 'The Specificity of Women's Sexual Response and Its Relationship with Sexual Orientations: A Review and Ten Hypotheses', *Archives of Sexual Behavior*, 46:1161–79 (2017).

5. Chivers, M.L. and Brotto, L.A., 'Controversies of Women's Sexual Arousal and Desire', *European Psychologist*, 22(1), 5–26 (2017).

6. Anderson, A.B. and Hamilton, L.D., 'Assessment of Distraction from Erotic Stimuli by Nonerotic Interference', *Journal of Sex Research*, 52:3, 317–26 (2015).

7. Beck, J.G. and Baldwin, L.E., 'Instructional Control of Female Sexual Responding', *Archives of Sexual Behavior*, 23(6), 665–84 (1994).

8. Silva, E., Pascoal, P.M. and Nobre, P., 'Beliefs about Appearance, Cognitive Distraction and Sexual Functioning in Men and Women: A Mediation Model Based on Cognitive Theory', *Journal of Sexual Medicine*, vol. 13 (9), 1387–94 (2016).

9. Janssen, E., Everaerd, W., Spiering, M. and Janssen, J., 'Automatic Processes and the Appraisal of Sexual Stimuli: Toward an Information Processing Model of Sexual Arousal', *Journal of Sex Research*, 37:1, 8–23 (2000).

10. Purdon, C. and Holdaway, L., 'Non-Erotic Thoughts: Content and Relation to Sexual Functioning and Sexual Satisfaction', *Journal of Sex Research*, 43(2), 154–62 (2006).

11. Laan, E. and Both, S., 'What Makes Women Experience Desire?', *Feminism and Psychology*, 18, 505–14 (2008); Toates, F.M., 'An Integrative Theoretical Framework for Understanding

Sexual Motivation, Arousal, and Behavior', *Journal of Sex Research*, 46:2–3, 168–93 (2009).

12. Solomon, R.L., 'The Opponent Process Theory of Motivation', *American Psychologist*, 35, 691–73 (1980).

13. Frederick, D.A., Lever, J., Gillespie, B.J. and Garcia, J.R., 'What Keeps Passion Alive? Sexual Satisfaction is Associated with Sexual Communication, Mood Setting, Sexual Variety, Oral Sex, Orgasm, and Sex Frequency in a National US Study', *Journal of Sex Research*, 54:2, 186–201 (2017).

14. Dewsbury, D.A., 'Effects of Novelty on Copulatory Behavior: The Coolidge Effect and Related Phenomena', *Psychological Bulletin*, 89, 464–82 (1981).

15. Sims, K.E. and Meana, M., 'Why Did Passion Wane? A Qualitative Study of Married Women's Attributions for Declines in Sexual Desire', *Journal of Sex & Marital Therapy*, 36(4), 360–80 (2010); Ferreira, L.C., Fraenkel, P., Narciso, I., and Novo, R., 'Is Committed Desire Intentional? A Qualitative Exploration of Sexual Desire and Differentiation of Self in Couples', *Family Process*, 54, 308–26 (2015).

16. Kabat-Zinn, J., *Full Catastrophe Living: How to Cope with Stress, Pain and Illness Using Mindfulness Meditation* (London: Piatkus, 1990).

17. Brotto, L.A., Seal, B.N. and Rellini, A., 'Pilot Study of a Brief Cognitive Behavioral versus Mindfulness-Based Intervention for Women with Sexual Distress and a History of Childhood Sexual Abuse', *Journal of Sex & Marital Therapy*, 38, 1–27 (2012); Velten, J., Margraf, J., Chivers, M.L. and Brotto, L.A., 'Effects of a Mindfulness Task on Women's Sexual Response', *Journal of Sex Research*, 55:6, 747–57 (2018); Gunst, A., Ventus, D., Arver, S., Dhejne, C., Görts-Öberg, K., Zamore-Söderström, E. and Jern, P., 'A Randomized, Waiting-List Controlled Study Shows that Brief, Mindfulness-Based Psychological Interventions are Effective for Treatment of Women's Low Sexual Desire', *Journal*

of Sex Research (2018).

18. Adam, F., Géonet, M., Day, J. and de Sutter, P., 'Mindfulness Skills are Associated with Female Orgasm?', *Sexual and Relationship Therapy*, 30:2, 256–67 (2015).

19. Wolkin, J.R., 'Cultivating Multiple Aspects of Attention through Mindfulness Meditation Accounts for Psychological Well-Being through Decreased Rumination', *Psychology Research and Behavior Management*, 8, 171–80 (2015).

20. Brotto, L.A., Basson, R., Smith, K.B., Driscoll, M. and Sadownik, L., 'Mindfulness-Based Group Therapy for Women with Provoked Vestibulodynia', *Mindfulness*, 6:417–32 (2015).

21. Kabat-Zinn, J., Lipworth, L. and Burney, R., 'The Clinical Use of Mindfulness Meditation for the Self-Regulation of Chronic Pain', *Journal of Behavioural Medicine*, 8, 163–90 (1985).

22. Brotto, L.A., *Better Sex through Mindfulness: How Women Can Cultivate Desire* (Vancouver, BC: Greystone Books, 2018).

7. Gaps in our understanding of desire

1. Laan, E. and Both, S., 'What Makes Women Experience Desire?', *Feminism and Psychology*, 18, 505–14 (2008); Basson, R., 'The Female Sexual Response: A Different Model', *Journal of Sex & Marital Therapy*, 26, 51–65 (2000).

2. Masters, W.H. and Johnson, V.E., *Human Sexual Response* (Boston, MA: Little Brown, 1966).

3. Kaplan, H.S., 'Hypoactive Sexual Desire', *Journal of Sex & Marital Therapy*, 3, 3–9 (1977).

4. Nowosielski, K., Wróbel, B. and Kowalczyk, R., 'Women's Endorsement of Models of Sexual Response: Correlates and Predictors', *Archives of Sexual Behavior*, 45, 291–302 (2016).

5. Bancroft, J. and Janssen, E., 'The Dual Control Model of Male Sexual Response: A Theoretical Approach to Centrally Mediated

Erectile Dysfunction', *Neuroscience and Biobehavioral Reviews*, 24, 571–79 (2000).

6. Nagoski, E., *Come as You Are: The Surprising New Science that Will Transform Your Sex Life* (London: Scribe Publications, 2015).

7. Sanders, S.A., Graham C.A. and Milhausen, R.R., 'Predicting Sexual Problems in Women: The Relevance of Sexual Excitation and Sexual Inhibition', *Archives of Sexual Behavior*, 37:241–51 (2008).

8. Basson, R., 'The Female Sexual Response: A Different Model', *Journal of Sex & Marital Therapy*, 26, 51–65 (2000); Basson, R., 'Using a Different Model for Female Sexual Response to Address Women's Problematic Low Sexual Desire', *Journal of Sex & Marital Therapy*, 27, 395–403 (2001).

9. Elaut, E., Buysse, A., De Sutter, P., Gerris, J., De Cuypere, G. and T'Sjoen, G., 'Cycle-Related Changes in Mood, Sexual Desire, and Sexual Activity in Oral-Contraception-Using and Nonhormonal-Contraception-Using Couples', *Journal of Sex Research*, 53:1, 125–36 (2016).

10. Mitchell, K.R., Geary, R., Graham, C.A., Datta, J., Wellings, K., Sonnenberg, P., Field, N., Nunns, D., Bancroft, J., Jones, K.G., Johnson, A.M. and Mercer, C.H., 'Painful Sex (Dyspareunia) in Women: Prevalence and Associated Factors in a British Population Probability Survey', *British Journal Obstetrics and Gynaecology*, 124:1689–97 (2017).

8. What next?

1. Carvalheira, A.A. and Leal, I.P., 'Masturbation among Women: Associated Factors and Sexual Response in a Portuguese Community Sample', *Journal of Sex & Marital Therapy*, 39, 347–67 (2012).

2. Laan, E., Everaerd, W., van Aanhold, M. and Rebel, M., 'Performance Demand and Sexual Arousal in Women',

Behaviour Research and Therapy, 31, 25–35 (1993).

3. McCarthy, B. and Wald, L.M., 'Strategies and Techniques to Directly Address Sexual Desire Problems', *Journal of Family Psychotherapy*, 26, 286–98 (2015).

4. De Shazer, S., *Keys to Solution in Brief Therapy* (New York, NY: Norton, 1985).

9. Futureproof your sex life, for life

1. Clark, M.S. and Mills, J.R., 'A Theory of Communal (and Exchange) Relationships' in Van Lange, P.A.M., Kruglanski, A.W., and Higgins, E.T. (eds.), *Handbook of Theories of Social Psychology* (Thousand Oaks, CA: Sage, 2012), vol. 2, pp. 232–50.

2. Mills, J.R., Clark, M. S., Ford, T.E. and Johnson, M., 'Measurement of Communal Strength', *Personal Relationships*, 11, 213–30 (2004).

3. Muise, A., Impett, E. A., Desmarais, S. and Kogan, A., 'Keeping the Spark Alive: Being Motivated to Meet a Partner's Sexual Needs Sustains Sexual Desire in Long-Term Romantic Relationships', *Social Psychological and Personality Sciences*, 4, 267–73 (2013).

4. Muise, A. and Impett, E.A., 'Good, Giving, and Game: The Relationship Benefits of Communal Sexual Motivation', *Social Psychological and Personality Sciences*, 6(2), 164–72 (2015); Muise, A., Impett, E.A., and Desmarais, S., 'Getting it On versus Giving It Up: Sexual Motivation, Desire, and Satisfaction in Intimate Bonds', *Personality and Social Psychology Bulletin*, 39, 1320–32 (2013); Muise, A., Impett, E. A., and Desmarais, S., 'Getting it On versus Giving It Up: Sexual Motivation, Desire, and Satisfaction in Intimate Bonds', *Personality and Social Psychology Bulletin*, 39, 1320 (2013).

5. McNulty, J.K. and Widman, L., 'The Implications of Sexual Narcissism for Sexual and Marital Satisfaction', *Archives of Sexual Behavior*, 42(6), 1021–32 (2013).

6. Velten, J., Brailovskaia, J. and Margraf, J., 'Exploring the Impact of Personal and Partner Traits on Sexuality: Sexual Excitation, Sexual Inhibition, and Big Five Predict Sexual Function in Couples', *Journal of Sex Research* (2018).

7. Aron, A. and Aron, E.N., *Love and the Expansion of Self: Understanding Attraction and Satisfaction* (New York, NY: Hemisphere, 1986).

8. Muise, A., Harasymchuk, C., Day, L.C., Bacev-Giles, C., Gere, J. and Impett, E. A., 'Broadening Your Horizons: Self-Expanding Activities Promote Desire and Satisfaction in Established Romantic Relationships', *Journal of Personality and Social Psychology* (2018).

9. Ferreira, L.C., Narciso, I., Novo, R.F. and Pereira, C.R., 'Predicting Couple Satisfaction: The Role of Differentiation of Self, Sexual Desire, and Intimacy in Heterosexual Individuals', *Sexual and Relationship Therapy*, 29, 390 (2014); Murray, S.H., Sutherland, O., and Milhausen, R.R., 'Young Women's Descriptions of Sexual Desire in Long-Term Relationships', *Sexual and Relationship Therapy*, 27, 3 (2012).

10. Lagaert, L., Weyers, S., Van Kerrebroeck, H. and Elaut, E., 'Postpartum Dyspareunia and Sexual Functioning: A Prospective Cohort Study', *European Journal of Contraception and Reproductive Health Care*, 22, 200–206 (2017); Wallwiener, S., Muller, M., Doster, A., Kuon, R.J., Plewniok, K., Feller, S., Wallwiener, M., Reck, C., Matthies, L.M., and Wallwiener, C., 'Sexual Activity and Sexual Dysfunction of Women in the Perinatal Period: A Longitudinal Study', *Archives of Gynecology and Obstetrics*, 295, 873–83 (2017).

11. Dosch, A., Ghisletta, P. and Van der Linden, M., 'Body Image in Dyadic and Solitary Sexual Desire: The Role of Encoding Style

and Distracting Thoughts', *Journal of Sex Research*, 53:9, 1193–206 (2016).

12. Forbes, M.K., Eaton, N.R. and Krueger, R.F., 'Sexual Quality of Life and Aging: A Prospective Study of a Nationally Representative Sample', *Journal of Sex Research*, 54(2):137–48 (2017); Hinchliff, S. and Gott, M., 'Challenging Social Myths and Stereotypes of Women and Ageing – Heterosexual Women Talk about Sex', *Journal of Women and Aging*, 20(1/2), 65–81 (2008).

Further Reading

Andrejek, N. and Fetner, T., 'The Gender Gap in Orgasms: Survey Data from a Mid-sized Canadian City', *International Journal of Sexual Health* (2019).

Brotto, L.A., Chivers, M.L., Millman, R.D. and Albert, A., 'Mindfulness-Based Sex Therapy Improves Genital-Subjective Arousal Concordance in Women with Sexual Desire/Arousal Difficulties', *Archives of Sexual Behavior*, 45, 1907–21 (2016).

Frost, R. and Donovan, C., 'A Qualitative Exploration of the Distress Experienced by Long-term Heterosexual Couples when Women Have Low Sexual Desire', *Sexual and Relationship Therapy* (2019).

Herbenick, D., Fu, T.C., Arter, J. and Sanders, S.A., 'Women's Experiences with Genital Touching, Sexual Pleasure, and Orgasm: Results from a US Probability Sample of Women Aged 18 to 94', *Journal of Sex & Marital Therapy*, 0 (0), 1–12 (2017).

Hendrickx, L., Gijs, L., and Enzlin, P., 'Who's Distressed by Sexual Difficulties? Exploring Associations between Personal, Perceived Partner, and Relational Distress and Sexual Difficulties in Heterosexual Men and Women', *Journal of Sex Research* (2018).

Impett, E.A., Muise, A. and Rosen, N.O., 'Is it Good to be Giving in the Bedroom? A Prosocial Perspective on Sexual Health and Well-being in Romantic Relationships', *Current Sexual Health Reports*, 7, 180–90 (2015).

Meana, M., 'Elucidating Women's (Hetero)Sexual Desire: Definitional Challenges and Content Expansion', *Journal of Sex Research*, 47:2–3, 104–22 (2010).

Murray, S.H., Milhausen, R.R., Graham, C.A. and Kuczynski, L., 'A Qualitative Exploration of Factors that Affect Sexual Desire among Men Aged 30 to 65 in Long-Term Relationships', *Journal of Sex Research*, 54:3, 319–30 (2017).

Salisbury, C.M.A. and Fisher, W.A., '"Did You Come?" A Qualitative Exploration of Gender Differences in Beliefs, Experiences and Concerns Regarding Female Orgasm Occurrence during Heterosexual Sexual Interactions', *Journal of Sex Research*, 51(6), 616–31 (2014).

Suschinsky, K.D., Huberman, J.S., Maunder, L., Brotto, L.A., Hollenstein, T. and Chivers, M.L., 'The Relationship between Sexual Functioning and Sexual Concordance in Women', *Journal of Sex and Marital Therapy* (2019).

Velten, J., Scholten, S., Graham, C.A., Adolph, D., and Margraf, J., *Archives of Sexual Behavior*, 45:1957–71 (2016).

Index

and variety 187
women who have sex with women
    83–6
see also satisfaction
Sexual Script Theory 80–6
sexual scripts 56–7, 80–91, 93, 108, 109,
    112, 146
  changing 269
  dominant 80–2
  and faking orgasms 96–7
  heterosexual 76–7, 83–4, 86, 94,
    94–9
  and initiation of sex 130–1
  media influence 86–9
  men and 92
  narrowness 101
  and oral sex 97–9
  pervasiveness 80
  and porn 89–91
  pressure from 214–15
  ramifications 82–3
  and reciprocity 97–9
  straight=best 85
  for women who have sex with
    women 83
sexual situation 61
sexual stimuli 167, 169, 170, 173, 190,
    208, 212, 228
  adequate 25
  and desire 214–15, 216–22, 232
  exercises 244–5
sexual trauma, impact of 188–9
sexual urges, fear of 14
sexuality 108
  change over lifetime 125, 256–7,
    257, 279–83
  changing needs 279–83
  connecting with 105
  control 16
  exploring 257–8
  influences on 257

relative value 153–9
  standards 1
Sexually Transmitted Infections 32
shame 14, 48, 176
sin 12–14, 18
skill 20
sleep deprivation 151
smartphones 149–50
social and cultural factors 75–112,
    124–5, 175, 287–8
  body image 99–100, 178, 279
  heteronormativity 83–4, 85–6, 86
  heterosexual 76–7
  importance of 91–4, 111
  internalized beliefs 76–7
  and intersectional identities 108–11
  language 100–3, 112
  learning about sex 79–86
  media influence 86–9, 109, 112
  porn 89–91, 112
  reflection 113–15
  sexual scripts 80–91, 94–9
  shifts over time 111
  social norms 77–9, 82
  unhelpful beliefs 103–7
social chat 31
social conditioning 132, 175
social control 15
social learning 79
social learning theory 184
social media 150, 179
social norms, role of 77–9, 82
social psychology 77–9, 80
social rules 82
socialization 98–9, 127, 166, 215
solo sex 66
spontaneous passion 88
spontaneous sex 148–9
  ease of 103–5
stimulation 62
strangers, sex with 118, 119